I0622205

Live Your Truth and Take Back Your Life (3 books in 1)

Stop Overthinking, Set Boundaries and Discover Self-Love.

Zera Young

Contents

Reframing Negative Thinking

Set Good Boundaries

The Proven Path to Self-Compassion

Get Your Ebook Stop Limiting Yourself
+ Reduce Stress in 1 minute [video]
+ Printable Gratitude Journal

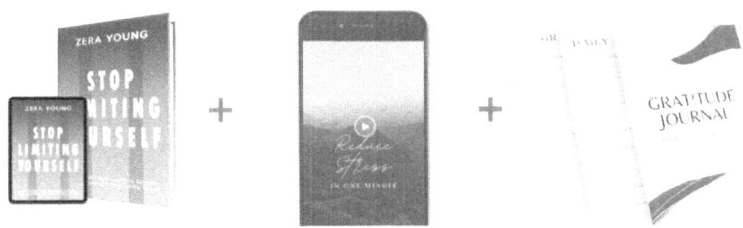

Scan the QR code below to claim your free bonuses
——————— OR ———————
visit gifts.zerayoung.com/bundle

Unleash your true potential and choose to live your best life!

✔ Free e-book: Stop Limiting Yourself. Stop doubting your potential and learn to recognize your self-limiting beliefs!

✔ Free meditation video: Reduce your stress levels in one minute with this powerful breathing exercise.

✔ Printable Journal: Print out your daily and monthly Personal Gratitude Journal for positive manifestation and improved self-confidence!

Reframing Negative Thinking

Transform Your Perspective, Calm Your Mind, Find Peace.

Introduction

When people ask me why I decided to write this book, they expect me to say that it's because of my expertise. In reality, I was just inspired to create something that will help people get out of their own way. I see kids in middle school or high school, already succumbing to the throes of negativity. In colleges and universities around the globe, we are seeing more and more young adults feeling lost, discouraged, and pessimistic about their futures. Later in life, these students grow into unhappy adults—stuck in a boring job and not even seeing the point of trying to escape. To them, it seems as if only the lucky ones become successful while the rest of us are forced deal with the innumerous adversities of life. Seeing so many young people not able to tap into their potential all because of the way their mind is wired, is what pushed me to create this book.

I have been divorced for nearly a decade now. I'm not going to lie to you, that period of my life was tough; I experienced a sense of loss, sadness, and grief, just like most other divorcees. What I realized through those emotions, however, was that I remained myself. I expected myself to shut down at some point, finding it unbearable to move on. To my pleasant surprise that expectation never came true. In fact, I soon found myself learning the difference between the feelings I was experiencing and the wonderful potential I had in my future; the people I had yet to meet and love, the countries I had yet to see and the languages I had yet to learn. My sadness didn't consume my being. I felt it, as you do with any loss, but it was separate from who I was. I looked forward to changing and experiencing my life in a whole new way. I had never felt more powerful in my life than at that moment. From this feeling sprouted my inspiration to help others feel this way.

Throughout my life, I used to be quite an influenceable person—I generally credit this to my previous people-pleasing tendency. As a child and teenager, I remember trying to conform to every new friend I made. Instead of finding who I was, I let others decide. Sad, isn't it? Even throughout college, I struggled to feel comfortable with myself. Between my family, friends, partners, and coworkers, I must have seemed like a different person to each. Through these types of attachments, I became vulnerable to their mindsets. I remember a particular boyfriend who made my life nearly unbearable—not because he was an abusive partner or anything, but rather because his constant pessimism rubbed off on me. I stopped setting high goals for myself, taking on challenges, and exploring myself. We both were lumps of disappointment. For over a year, I felt miserable while being unaware of the reason. Slowly, I began to notice that when I would take trips with my friends away from my then-boyfriend, I felt different. At first, I was confused. After all, we were supportive of each other, and if I ever felt bad about something or myself, he was there for me. Yet, here I was, watching myself put my own spark out. Eventually, I realized that the support we were offering each other was only confirming our disappointment in the world. We listened, talked, discussed, but failed to uplift each other. We fed into loops of negativity that only further reinforced our beliefs that the world was a bad place where bad things were bound to happen. Within a month or two after coming to that conclusion, I found a way to respectfully end things and saw the difference that being alone made.

Through single life, boyfriends, and ex-husbands, I have seen it all. I realize now that having good people around you is important, but nothing will ever top being good to yourself. We will feel alone at times, no matter how hard we try not to. It is how we handle being by ourselves that can show us the true measure of our relationship with ourselves. Are we kind to ourselves? Do we put too much pressure on ourselves? Do we belittle our accomplishments?

There are many, many ways one can make life hell for themselves. Sadly, this is a natural route for a large majority of the population. Without unlearning these things, we will stay harmful toward ourselves and potentially others.

I've always believed that the world had too much to offer for so many people to not let themselves experience it. Word by word, I want to help you and anyone else who comes across this book to take the power back from negativity—and not through commonly overused phrases mask your sadness. You can do this through advice that will actually change your life bit by bit.

"You don't have it that bad!"

"You should be grateful for what you've got."

"Just change your mindset—be positive!"

We've all heard this so-called advice. However, no one seems to explain *how* we should accomplish these things. Psychology and mindset are extremely complex issues. They have to do with emotions, neurology, physical lifestyle, and life history. That's why it's so hard to come up with a solution that can work for everyone. So, instead of doing that, I will be providing you with extremely applicable basics of transforming your negative thoughts into more constructive ones. There is no one-size-fits-all, but there are different options available.

Chapter 1
Understanding Negative Thinking

"Dwelling on the negative simply contributes to its power."

— *Shirley MacLaine*

The first thing you need to know is that your brain is technically wired to think negatively. Originally, this wiring served as a defense mechanism —one that dates back to the dawn of mankind, when people were cavemen and cavewomen with only a few main objectives: hunt and scavenge for food and protect themselves, and their offspring, from danger. If you think the world is a dangerous place now, imagine what it was like back then, with none of the amenities or safety measures we have today. The average caveman had to be wary of savage beasts and, well, savage fellow cavemen. Nowadays, modern society is practically built on businesses that have found a way to simplify and make life more pleasant. As if restaurants were not good enough of an idea, we now have food delivery services. The objectives of an average person are now multiplied. With safety and food accounted for (for the most part), we now busy ourselves with other things. We worry about promotions and learning to play an instrument and being environmentally friendly.

Again, this was not what people worried about in the past. With food and safety being their primary concerns, the brains of primitive humans began accommodating these needs. Their brains learned to be extra aware of the numerous dangers that posed a threat to their lives, and their negative appreciation of said dangers is what kept them alive.

Although most of these dangers are no longer as prevalent in the contemporary age, that negative thought mechanism has managed to persist, being handed down from generation to generation, like getting an inheritance that is more of a burden than a gift. At least, that is how we perceive it now, right? But what if we started seeing it as a gift once again; a gift that we often mismanage and fail to have control over, but a gift nonetheless. Negative thoughts are meant to serve a purpose. It is through a lack of knowledge and experience we fail to see them for the beneficial tendencies they are. In reality, negative thoughts continue to be useful for us—and often life-saving.

For early humans, assuming something unfamiliar is life-threatening could determine whether they lived or died. If they came across an unfamiliar berry, they would be risking their offspring's lives if they assumed it was harmless and fed it to them. Instead, these people would have assumed the worst and decided their course of action from there. Nowadays, we apply a similar logic, but to much less drastic situations. We might be afraid of asking someone out, thinking that they'll reject us immediately and we'll never recover. Similar assumptions, right? Yet, one seemed to protect the person, while the other kept them from taking an innocent risk. With examples like these, it becomes quite clear that negativity is not the villain we make it out to be. Rather, we just have the responsibility of learning how to use and apply it.

Our Place in the Modern World

There seems to have been more than one pandemic in recent history. One involves a life-threatening virus that has traveled around the globe, while the other is found in people's mindsets. One can argue that living in the Paleolithic era of humanity, hunting and scavenging for food is the worst life imaginable. This is probably true for most people who enjoy sleeping in a nice bed, taking hot showers, and exchanging currency for prepared foods and other ingredients. However, in a lot of ways, one might romanticize the simplicity of the past; not necessarily the dawn of humanity, but let's say a few hundred years back. Nowadays, we seem to be faced with a new type of technology every few months, falling behind on trends, and never having time to do everything we want. The world has been far from perfect, with the present included. Modern society has its fair share of wonderful additions, while, in turn, making other aspects of our lives pay for them.

In my everyday life, I come across so many people who are lost. They don't know why they're doing what they're doing or even whether they want to be doing it at all. As many as 44% of undergraduate students don't know what they want to be doing after they graduate from university (Concrete, 2022). Of course, some people's reactions might be disbelief, while others may blame these students for being so out of touch with their desires. But is it really their fault?

In most countries around the world, students are asked to pick a field of study, in which they will have to invest a lot of money, at the young age of 18. A few lucky ones might know what they want to study, while the rest are left struggling to make such a crucial choice. If they choose 'wrong', they may end up spending years of their young lives and thousands of dollars on an education they neither needed nor desired. So, many begin to contemplate this choice based on factors other than true desire, including: how much money they can make from this degree, how hard it is to get into the program, and how the people around them will perceive them with such a degree. Even without a true calling for their choice of program, they might carry on studying it for years, getting a degree, and even becoming a professional in that field before realizing their life doesn't truly belong to them. Being in your 30s, 40s, or even older, and realizing that you've been living a life based on somebody else's criteria is a terrifying realization but not an uncommon one. For many reasons, these poor students are not to blame. Instead, the root of the issue lies in the way our society is organized and the immense pressure that is put upon the shoulders of these young adults.

A similar phenomenon follows us into later adulthood, where the same concept is applied: we make lifestyle choices that we *think* will make us happy based on someone else's standards. Hustle culture is a fantastic example of a modern mindset that has managed to decrease the quality of life for millions of people, while pretending to do quite the opposite. If you aren't already familiar with this term, hustle culture can be defined as the belief that true happiness and success come to those who spend as much time as possible being productive and earning money. Not only does this philosophical trend leave no time for rest for the affected individuals, but its true benefit is not to the individual—it's to capitalism. We have somehow managed to convince ourselves that over-working our bodies and minds like some lab rats is the true definition of prosperity.

In many cultures and religions around the world, the idea of hustle culture would be laughed at. Thanks to many Eastern beliefs that emphasize the importance of balance and calmness, this phenomenon would not have made it past the fame of a niche Facebook group. And yet, here so many of us are acting as if working for 90 hours per week is something worth bragging about. Why do we use our exhaustion as a measure of social status? Too many of us fail to listen to ourselves, and instead take advice from people who may not have our best interests in mind.

Negativity: A Cultural Phenomenon?

Let's take a look around the world: How do different countries' and cultures' happiness levels compare? Well, some of you may or may not be surprised to know that Nordic countries are among the happiest in the world. In 2019, Finland scored highest on happiest, followed by Denmark, Norway, Iceland, and eventually Sweden in seventh place (Bloom, 2022). Their taxes are higher than in the United States, for example, yet the average Finn is much happier than the average American. Not surprisingly, Nordic countries also tend to score highest in quality of life; this pertains to education, social welfare, healthcare, access to necessities, etcetera. Just to mention a few wonderful differences, these countries have strict laws that guarantee adequate maternal and paternal leave, a humane prison system focused on rehabilitation, and tax distribution that allows citizens to trust their social security. Unfortunately, the same can rarely be said for much of the United States, where happiness has been *declining*. Prices in the US are rising exponentially while income is not—can this be the reason we're so unhappy? The statistical comparison of quality of life and happiness between North America and Northern Europe sure seems to suggest so, but it isn't the *only* reason.

Ikigai Is Key

In Japan, there exists an ancient philosophy called Ikigai. Ikigai is often regarded as a source of someone's life purpose or reason for living. This philosophy and way of life is often used as part of the reason why people living in the blue zone of Okinawa Japan have such a high life expectancy. A National Geographic explorer, Dan Buettner, recorded a stone inscription he found in Okinawa, Japan—"At 80, you are merely a youth. At 90, if your ancestors invite you into heaven, ask them to wait until you are 100—then, you might consider it" (Goss, 2020). In the entire world, there are currently five identified blue zones in which people are living the longest and are generally very healthy. These zones have been the subject of many scientific and philosophical studies, and the insights provided by their citizens can teach the rest of us a lot.

Okinawans have commonly suggested the following factors of their lives as the reasons for their health and longevity:

- **Having a sense of purpose.** As I described at the beginning of this chapter, our fast-paced lives in the West often shift our focus from purpose to productivity. We fail to ask ourselves: What is the point of productivity if it has no purpose? Among other populations, work-life balance is not treated as an afterthought, but rather, as a priority. Through Ikigai, people make finding their purpose a central focus of their time because they believe this is what grants them their good health and long lives. The practice of developing a sense of purpose has a lot to do with *why* we feel our emotions and not just *what* we are feeling. This demands a lot of introspection and resistance to shying away from what you might uncover when you examine yourself more deeply.

- **Deep focus and dedication.** As said, Ikigai adds purpose to people's actions. This, in turn, gives them the ability to focus on their tasks with much more ease than the average person. Knowing that what they are tasked with doing is benefitting their life's purpose, they have no problem mustering up enough concentration that would shock the average, Western procrastinator. Developing focus on things that matter is said to be a crucial aspect of improving your relationship with your life's purpose. To do so, I would recommend starting slow; challenge yourself to work on something you've been putting off for 15 to 30 minutes per day. If it's something that has any value to you, you will start to notice that this allotted time becomes easier and easier to stick to. The true challenge of improving your focus is to trust yourself enough to start.

- **Maintaining physical health.** In Okinawa, the key to longevity stems beyond purpose and focus. In fact, many Okinawans emphasize the crucial relationship between physical and mental health. Without physical health it is difficult to maintain good mental health, and without proper mental health it is difficult to stick to healthy eating and exercise regimens. We often associate diet and exercise with losing weight or building muscle mass, but its effects envelop much more of the human body. Neurologically, our brains have been found to release feel-good hormones following a workout that are capable of uplifting our moods for up to 24 hours afterward. Not surprisingly, staying active daily is a commitment many Okinawans partake in. They also report following the 80% rule—only eating until you feel 80% full to avoid being drained by overeating. A lot of Okinawans eat a largely vegetable-based diet with only a few meat products, if any at all.

- **Having a strong, supportive network.** The term "moai" refers to a dedicated friend group that supports one another for nearly an entire lifetime. It is this social network that provides people with adequate socialization, authentic companionship, and the option to receive true emotional and mental support. These aspects are important to everyone's emotional processing, and positively impact the way we manage difficult situations and feelings. Through moai, Okinawans receive all of these great benefits that help them stay mentally and emotionally satisfied. Now, like most people, you may not get to experience the stability of a moai, but the underlying lesson is that having people you can lean on from time to time isn't something to overlook; it truly improves your quality of life.

The Dark Side of Technology

Social media is complicated. I'm not one to bash the progress that we have made with technology, but I am one to notice its flaws. Social media was initially made to facilitate our interactions with people all around the globe. This made travel and moving away much easier for billions of people and was, put simply, a great invention. However, the dark side of social media did not wait long to manifest. As humans, it is normal for us to feel proud of ourselves. Furthermore, we want *others* to confirm this feeling and be proud of us as well. Many people believe that the need for external validation is a bad thing, but it isn't; it's a normal desire, and we can never truly get rid of every ounce of it. But, scrolling through social media we see a very different end of this spectrum. We come across dozens, hundreds, if not thousands of posts per week whose *only* purpose is external validation. There is no getting around it: social media can easily make a person feel bad about themselves or their life if they give it the power to do so. Seeing extravagant vacations, five-star dinners, and cars that cost as much as our houses will unavoidably have a negative effect on our mindset. Suddenly, the life we might have been satisfied with previously seems like nothing in comparison to the glamorous glimpses we see of other people.

Comparison is a dangerous tendency of ours. Just like negativity, comparison has beneficial roots. In other words, it benefitted us as cavepeople in a similar fashion: If you saw a fellow caveman get three times as many berries as you, your tendency to compare would probably push you to find out how they managed to do so. However, when the things we begin comparing become superficial or simply luxurious, our reactions brew toxicity. Not only do we become vulnerable to jealousy, envy, and hostility, our gratitude for what we *do* have automatically decreases—and suddenly, nothing is enough.

Rejecting the Herd

There's a contradiction in Western society that contributes to our happiness, or lack thereof. Unlike many cultures found in the Eastern parts of the world, our society is very individualistic rather than collectivist; meaning, we each tend to focus on our independence more than on the interconnectivity of society. Some even find this tendency to be a little cold to others, breeding a lack of trust within the population. However, even with all this individuality, we still often struggle to take our own paths.

When someone chooses to be themselves—in whatever capacity that may be—it is still regarded as a brave choice. This leads us to the discovery that individuality in modern society is solely about independence rather than an embrace of uniqueness; you get rewarded for not depending on others, but still punished for challenging the standards set by society.

Although there has been a slight decrease in this in the past decade or so, the choice many young adults make to not go to college, for example, is still regarded as a bad one. With insurmountable university fees, this choice seems like a no-brainer to many people. But, to society, this choice is not a celebrated one. You have to be strong in order to make a choice that doesn't make most people happy, even if it only affects you.

No wonder that with this psychology, so many people simply make choices to appease others.

The Effects of Negativity

If I were to ask each reader of this book to create a pros and cons list of negativity, I would expect to see a disequilibrium between the two; most people see negativity as a thing they want to get rid of.

The benefits of negativity are certainly present but get overshadowed by the innumerous drawbacks. For example, negativity can prevent us from getting hurt by something in the future, such as getting rejected from a job we wanted. On the other hand, the same negativity can prevent us from getting exactly what we want in the future, such as being hired for that job we really wanted. Our negativity is a double-edged sword, and we act according to which side we think we will regret the least. Most people in society are risk-averse, meaning they prefer to take smaller risks and as infrequently as possible. This group is most likely to not apply for their dream job at all because they believe the possibility of rejection is not worth the possibility of acceptance. Why is that?

An interesting psychological phenomenon explains why. People are notoriously bad at predicting our future emotional reactions. We overestimate both potential happiness and potential sadness. For instance, imagine how you would feel about getting your dream car or house. In your mind, you are likely to think your life will feel just a little more complete and that the happiness from this purchase will fill many voids, in turn increasing your life's overall quality. However, in reality, the happiness from such a purchase tends to wear off pretty quickly and completely fails to satisfy the buyer long-term. The same is applied to situations of sadness; we will predict that being rejected from a job will crush us and demotivate us for a very long time, which is simply not true. Much like the happiness from a luxurious purchase, the sadness from an event wears off as well. This phenomenon is called *impact bias* and is relevant to most people. Winning the lottery doesn't mean life-long happiness just as much as experiencing an unfortunate accident doesn't mean lifelong sadness. Convincing ourselves otherwise leads to dissatisfaction and only brews more negativity.

As true as it is that negativity also brings benefits, let's focus on why you don't want too much of it. After all, why else would you be reading this book? So, to examine why reframing negative thinking is an unavoidable task for happiness, let's take a look at what life would look like if you didn't.

Self-Esteem and Confidence

Negativity provides easy access to answering the unknown. What I mean by this, is that it offers us an idea of how something might turn out, and therefore becomes easy to overuse. Rather than wonder how we might look in a certain outfit, negativity allows us to find an answer: bad. Clearly, the downside to having the answer is that that answer will fail to be positive.

When there is too much negativity, it starts applying itself to everything —your career, your appearance, your skills, the outcomes of your risks, etcetera. Self-esteem and confidence are no exceptions, either. Someone with too much negativity will inevitably focus on the bad of something more than they realize the good of it. This also applies to themselves. They will often underestimate their skills and overestimate their flaws. While walking through a crowded place, they might feel exceptionally self-conscious regarding a small issue with their wardrobe that others will likely not even notice. Negativity causes them to pick and pick at themselves until they feel unworthy of success.

This low self-esteem and low confidence consequently cause a decrease in motivation. If everything will fail, what's the point of even trying? The person slowly becomes more and more risk-averse until taking chances doesn't seem worth it whatsoever. If they don't break out of this mindset, it soon consumes all their potential. Their dreams, their goals, their desire—all of these will be no match to the scary potential outcomes that negativity has spewed out. These things will not be sought after, making them irrelevant to the individual's life.

Avoiding this outcome requires either luck or effort. Either you're lucky enough to never get sucked into this vortex in the first place or you make a commitment to actively fight against it. Your mind is more powerful than the things that influence it. Negativity is not your whole mind; it is simply a mindset—and the great thing about mindsets is that they can definitely be changed.

Key Points

Let's look over the most important takeaways from Chapter 1:

- Negativity is not innately bad and can be quite beneficial
- Negativity in the modern world has become overwhelming
- Our perception of the world is influenced by our environment
- Ikigai teaches the importance of finding purpose
- Choosing to reject society's influence of negativity is a radical step
- Too much negativity affects your life and your perception of yourself

Chapter 2
Psychology and Philosophy Over the Years

"History is the interpretation of the significance that the past has for us."

— Johan Huizinga

The quote above will make sense in a moment, as in the chapter, we are learning from our past as a society. But first, let me tell you why this is significant. When I first got divorced, I jotted down a list of things I was eager to finally do. It's not like I couldn't have done them while I was still married, but something felt as if it was holding me back—until I got divorced. I used to be 'smarter' about my money. I think I was even a little too cautious. At one point I may have forgotten that money is meant to be spent, yet all the while I saved for a house and car that were still years away on my timeline. When I became single once again, I eventually dedicated a good part of my paycheck to travel. One year I went to South America, another I visited some countries in Asia, then I went to see a college friend in Northern Europe—these were truly revitalizing experiences, one after another. In all honesty, I have no intention of stopping. I have found what makes me appreciate my life and I will not apologize for enjoying it as much as I do.

The purpose of these trips, however, does not meet its end on my Instagram feed. Yes, I do it largely for the thrill it gives me, but I take home much more than a few pretty pictures and a souvenir. Thanks to my various adventures, I have learned more from them than I did from the first 35 years of my life.

Following my divorce, the first place I traveled to was Brazil. I had a friend in my late 20s who was infatuated with this country and later met a serious boyfriend there. She kept inviting me to go with her on her trips, but I often found excuses not to—I was intimidated. With my divorce came my newfound sense of adventure, and that intimidation disappeared.

When I got to Brazil, I understood why she fell in love with it. She was an attractive person, not just physically, but energetically; Brazil reflected these characteristics just the same. I have never been too much into the party scene and was quite cautious when it came to the Amazon Rainforest, so I spent my time exploring the culture. I visited museum after museum, as well as many landmarks, and lots of other things you could find on the first two pages of Yelp suggestions. My trip didn't end there, however, as I found myself in Peru next. Here, the most popular destination is evidently the famous Machu Picchu; but, even after visiting such exquisite sites, I didn't feel fully satisfied.

Fast forward a few weeks and I was finally comfortable. Or rather, I was comfortable being uncomfortable. I was still equally nervous striking up conversations with random people, but I managed to stop looking at Yelp and began interacting with the locals as best as I could (Google Translate certainly helped). Every city and country I visited afterward, I did the same—I started being less interested in the tourist attractions and more focused on learning from the people. I could tell countless stories and recount endless conversations that have all shaped me into who I am today, but all I will say is this: There is so much we do not know.

Only through dozens, if not hundreds, of people had I learned so much. They told me stories of their families and traditions, invited me to dinner, showed me around neighborhoods, and so much more that opened my eyes to ways of life I had never even considered. It is from these interactions that I realized how crucial broadening our knowledge is; not just about facts and statistics, but about people and cultures.

Negativity is born from many things. Some are environmental, and some are from repeated choices, but the trends indicating that some cultures tend to be happier than others are not a coincidence. It is my solid belief that learning how philosophies and ways of life fluctuate between cultures and time periods can make it so much easier for us to change our perspectives. If you are truly interested in creating a mindset for yourself that will benefit your success, I can only recommend you have a basic knowledge of this information. In fact, by seeing the changes in mindset that occur throughout the world's history makes us realize that standards change. If you don't like the mentality that has been cultivated around you, you don't have any obligation to follow it.

Ancient Times

Even without doing any research, most people are probably aware of how drastically the world has changed over the past few thousand years. This change has not only regarded technology and medicine, but even just the way we tend to think. Witnessing someone being burned at the stake or decapitated in public is an unthinkable event nowadays, but in the past it might have been a fun Friday night for some people. This level of violence is insane to think about for us, but back then it was not something most people were extremely affected by. Were they simply born with characteristics that better equipped them for this lifestyle or were they influenced by their environments? How about surgeons or soldiers, even in the modern day? Some people I know would rather break an arm than get poked with a needle, while others spend 50+ hours a week cutting people open. There must be some aspects of this that are innate, while others are certainly products of the way we grow up.

A lot of people associate the far past with violence, pain, war, and so on. Most of us can't even imagine living 100 years ago, let alone 500 or 2,000. However, I'd argue that this completely overlooks the wonderful things that arose during that time. In fact, in a lot of ways, life back then was a lot more peaceful.

The Influence of Hinduism and Buddhism

Two years after my South American trip, I finally made it to Asia. I had been once before to Japan as a young teenager, accompanying my father on a brief business trip, and I had been longing to go back ever since. Fast forward 20-something years and I finally got to go again.

I probably don't have to tell you that Asia and its multitude of diverse cultures is an absolute gem. No, I don't mean the Asia that some people in the West may just assume refers to China, Japan, and Korea. I mean the Asia that also includes rural Thailand, the beaches of Indonesia, gorgeous Indian markets, and countless other countries. We often limit our knowledge of a place and time to what we are shown. In the West, most of Asian culture that we have access to comes from East Asia, which is why people's knowledge beyond China, Japan, and Korea tends to be quite restricted. But what if we ventured beyond those?

During my trip to Asia as an adult, I visited several countries. For the relevance of this chapter, however, I will focus on India. This wonderful Southeast Asian country has so much to offer, I'd need ten books the size of this one to even scratch the surface of what I've learned. Its rich culture and history have some of the oldest origins known to man, with several religions making up the bulk of its population's beliefs.

Hinduism is one of the oldest religions that we are aware of. In fact, when the Hindu *Vedas* (collections of religious texts) were written between 1500 and 1200 BCE, Hinduism had already existed for quite some time. The religion has existed for more than 3,500 years and remains relevant in today's world, with over 1 billion followers globally. So, what about this religion is continuing to attract so many people?

Hinduism has a main objective: escape *samsara*—the cycle of death and rebirth—through the accumulation of good *karma*—the energy of a person's past actions. This objective is called *moksha*. In this religion, there exists an ultimate, supreme being that is often referred to as Brahman. Oftentimes, this being is represented by hundreds of different deities. The appearance of so many gods and goddesses often leads people to think of Hinduism as a polytheistic religion, but that tends to be misrepresented.

Unlike Hinduism, Buddhism is slightly newer and does not have a supreme being, but did also originate in India. Around 500 BCE, a man named Siddartha Guatama (later known as the Buddha) first reached enlightenment. Buddhism has several overlaps with Hinduism—it also possesses the main objective of escaping reincarnation, which is also called samsara. This is also accelerated through the buildup of good karma, however, there is a better way of doing so. In Buddhism, there exists the concept of *nirvana* or spiritual enlightenment that connects the individual so strongly to the other realm that they don't need to be reincarnated again. Similarly to Hinduism, Buddhism continues to interest a lot of people around the world and currently has around 500 million followers.

The reason I gave you a quick overview of these religions is to introduce you to something I found particularly interesting while learning about Buddhism: In this particular belief system, Buddhists are urged to follow the *Middle Way*. This concept teaches the importance of balance. Instead of trying to reach a state of enlightenment through having too much or too little, people should strive to have just enough balance for a comfortable life, but not anything of excess. Why I found this so interesting is because several other religions often believe that worldly possessions are vain because our spirits and/or souls don't need them. I found a connection between the concept of the Middle Way and the approach I used to maintain my mental health in good condition. Too much of something can be as bad as too little of something, and vice versa—and this applies to negativity.

Mindfulness From Zen Buddhism

A branch of Buddhism called Zen Buddhism happens to focus on a person's mindset and lifestyle. It centers around the cultivation of peace and calmness, not only through one's thinking, but by changing their surroundings to facilitate this process. This is also something that I have found useful for my own life: The way we live, the habits we form, and the actions we make all contribute to forming our mindsets. Buddhism, Hinduism, and particularly Zen Buddhism, all promote mindfulness.

Mindfulness is a state of mind that is meant to make us aware of our present. It is often applied to all areas of life, including how we eat, how we focus, what we say, etcetera. Mindful eating is a popular approach to cultivating a healthy diet, through attentiveness. This would look like paying special attention to what you are consuming: how does it taste? What are its colors? How would you describe the texture?

Mindfulness is believed to promote a calm mind—one in which there are no obstacles to enjoying the moment. Rather than focusing on stressing about the future or regretting the past, mindfulness brings us to this very moment; it quiets the mind and allows us to stop being influenced by pestering thoughts. This might be one of the best ways to stop letting negativity take over.

15th to 19th Centuries

It's quite impossible to capture all of the cultural changes that occurred around the world in five whole centuries that may have influenced the population's mindset, but we can focus on important trends. When we look at the way people's approaches to life have changed from the 15th to 19th centuries, we are making a big generalization. After all, there were always outliers and major differences between different places in the world, making it difficult to find a common average.

As we look at the overview of each era, we begin to realize the patterns. Oftentimes, we can directly see a connection between societal standards and expectations, and the mindset people had at that time.

Renaissance Era

The Renaissance Era lasted between the 14th and 17th centuries. Unlike the Middle Ages, which came directly before—often characterized as dark and centered largely around survival from various dangers—the Renaissance Era is known for promoting classical art, music, and philosophy. Suddenly, the world became a little less dark with a lot more beauty. This era produced some of the most famous and intricate works of art and music. The word "renaissance" even means "rebirth" in French, symbolizing this colossal transformation in the Western European world.

One huge product of the Renaissance Era is humanism—a strong intellectual movement that encouraged people to focus on being human. Rather than doing everything out of a religious or survival need, humanism brought to light the importance of savoring our lives. This, in turn, was captured in the impressive works of art during this era.

Beyond just art, humanism also wanted people to take responsibility for their actions and morals outside of religion. It promoted a person's autonomous contribution to society in a way that put people and society first and religion second. Humanism emphasized the need for education to become a priority in order for people to learn how to be a good person before they learn how to be a good follower of religion.

This was a relatively drastic shift—no wonder it took up to three centuries! The mindset had suddenly shifted from mostly just honoring God and trying to survive to enjoying what it means to be human and educating oneself. Furthermore, people slowly began seeing each other as more valuable. If beforehand other people were simply followers of God, now they were more likely to be seen as equally important creations by God, and warranted more respect. People focused more on individuality and were allowed some degree of uniqueness finally. It is difficult to say definitively, but due to the Renaissance Era being regarded as the transition from darkness into a lighter time, it makes sense to assume that this era brought a more optimistic point of view.

Age of Enlightenment

In the 17th century, there came a new philosophical and intellectual movement—the Enlightenment. Here, the focus became rationality. The whirlwind of art, music, and philosophical literature was replaced by scientific discoveries and bold new ideas. Suddenly, people were focused on finding explanations for things outside of religion and art. Rather than thinking about what it means to be human-like in the previous era—people wanted answers to questions such as: Does the universe work without the influence of God? How do we rationally explain certain phenomena? What if we organized society with human well-being at the center and not religious ruling?

It was a tumultuous time and, most likely, not a much happier one than the Renaissance Era. However, these turbulent changes played a critical role in the development of society through the coming centuries, indicating a very strong shift in society's approach to life. People were finally waking up and getting the courage to fight back against the regimes that had been imposed on them. This era marks one of the most powerful examples of people breaking free from standards they were expected to simply accept. For example, writer Mary Wollstonecraft wrote *A Vindication of the Rights of Woman* in 1792, becoming an important icon in early feminism she sprouted from the changes exhibited throughout this era. Many people started thinking outside the box, questioning established routines, and encouraging people to think for themselves.

Can you identify the influence that the Age of Enlightenment has had on the modern world? Without these trailblazers, we would most likely have been far behind in societal progress. They paved the way for fighting for a better life and being proud of one's own beliefs. Although we still often face backlash from speaking our minds against societal standards, it is now much less of a taboo topic to discuss with others.

These changes are directly responsible for people's escape from lifestyles that didn't allow them to be happy and helped them stop being afraid to do so. Although negativity was probably *heightened* throughout this era due to people focusing on the bad so that they could fix it, it is a prime example of *good* negativity; negativity that lifts people up, rather than brings them down, which is a powerful mechanism for positive change.

Romanticism

The Romanticism Era is a direct product of the Enlightenment, but is considerably shorter than most of the previously examined eras, lasting roughly between 1800 and 1850. For this time period, society makes a return to celebrating life: art, music, literature, education, etcetera. But this time, we take it a step further. Rather than examining human life outside of religion, the focus was now on individualism itself. The forward-thinking fighters of the Enlightenment Era are the ones to thank for this.

Whereas the Age of Enlightenment centered around rationality and materials, Romanticism preferred the more subjective aspects of life. Individualism in the period of Romanticism allowed people to examine their emotions. The dust had slightly settled on fighting for freedom, and now, people were fighting for immaterial values.

People were finally allowed to feel and express their emotions with less opposition. They explored their beliefs deeper and were slightly more free to find ones that suited them better. They created art that reflected their passion and thought imagination was the best source of creation.

Aspects of Romanticism can quite clearly be seen today, with the recent increase in concern regarding mental health and emotional wellbeing reflecting this. It's not difficult, nowadays, to run into a person who proudly expresses their emotions through art, and that's truly a great thing to see. This period of Romanticism brought forth an important philosophy that continues to be relevant today: Don't ignore the more complicated and abstract parts of being human—express them.

Key Points

Let's look over the most important takeaways from Chapter 2:

- Understanding different approaches to life across time periods should inspire us to take our power back and not rely on the world to control our perceptions
- Society fluctuates between different perceptions of life
- Negativity is treated very differently across various cultures
- Changes in politics, the economy, and social security strongly influence our relationship with ourselves and our negative perception
- Trends exhibited in the past are key to our journey to positivity today

Chapter 3
Types of Negative Thinking

"Most misunderstandings in the world could be avoided if people would simply take the time to ask, 'What else could this mean?'"

— *Shannon L. Alder*

There's one reason why stopping negative thoughts tends to be so difficult: There are so many of them. Not only that, but even the term "negative thinking" is so broad, it encapsulates many different types. Negativity does not have only one form. Tackling all of them is what makes this task so challenging for many people.

Why Does Everything Seem So Bad?

You are obviously aware of the fact that your mind's negativity may be badly influencing your life, but are there perhaps some forms of negative thinking that you engage in without even realizing it? In this chapter, we'll be looking into what scientists call "cognitive distortions," which are essentially ways in which people perceive what happens around them in a distorted and negative manner. Such thoughts usually occur as incorrect assumptions, unrealistic self-criticisms, or even the denial of reality; and yet, their effects on you can often go unnoticed. When those thoughts start forming patterns, they become cognitive distortions—a term used to describe a person's inaccurate perception of reality. These cognitive distortions may then cause a person to believe false things about themselves or their place in the world, leading to various mental health issues.

Learning to recognize those cognitive distortions can help you avoid them and prevent them from leading to bad outcomes. Typical cognitive distortions include believing you are unworthy of success, thinking everyone sees you as lazy or incompetent or blaming yourself for the end of a relationship.

Examples of Negative Thinking

<u>Catastrophizing</u>

As the name indicates, catastrophizing occurs when we blow an issue out of proportion, making us react with a disproportionate level of emotion. This can often happen when we are already experiencing difficult emotions prior to the issue occurring. Being in a bad mood already makes us predisposed to seeing other things as worse than they are. However, catastrophizing can also originate from the issue itself, no matter how small it may be in reality. For many people, it may be because they have that reaction as a default setting—bad things seem *very* bad, and good things receive an underwhelming reaction. Let me give you an example: My mother was truly a light in my life, but the older I got, the more flaws I saw in her mentality at times; she was a worrier. She worried about me, she worried about my dad, she worried about her clients, and so on. When something bad would occur—as small as me having to delay my visit to her by a few days—it would be enough to ruin her mood for a week. On the other hand, her reaction to good surprises didn't meet the same fate—her happiness didn't last nearly as long.

I loved my mother with all my heart, and when I became old enough for her to fully trust me, she let me help her. I offered suggestions on how she can experience happiness more fully and sadness less invasively, and eventually we saw some progress. To make her feel less alone, I often participated in the exercises. When something bad would happen to us, we would answer the following questions together:

- What is my initial go-to reaction to this issue?
- Was this issue truly preventable by me or not?
- Will this issue affect me badly in one week, one month, or one year from now?
- Is there anything I can do going forward to make myself feel better?
- What have I learned from this issue, if anything?

With enough repetition, my mother's initial reaction of catastrophizing was slowly replaced by answering these questions. Suddenly, analyzing the issue through this lens was her new, go-to reaction.

Overgeneralization

Let's say you're a teacher. It's the end of the semester and the students submit their feedback on your performance. One student said you failed to explain things clearly enough, so they ended the semester more confused than they had started it. Instead of accepting the feedback and vowing to be clearer going forward, you take it to heart, and start thinking, "I'm a terrible teacher." Even if feedback from the rest of the class was positive, you still fixate on that one comment and apply it to your entire performance, to your whole career—you are a terrible teacher and that's that.

Not too helpful, is it? This is how overgeneralization operates—it makes us fixate on one singular detail, overlooking the abundance of others. This one tiny thing is given far too much importance and can become the entire way we view ourselves. Rather than acknowledging that we all have strengths and weaknesses, we analyze ourselves only through the context of that one pesky, disappointing detail.

You may ask, then: What is the difference between catastrophizing and overgeneralizing? Both of them take small things and blow them out of proportion, right? The difference is that catastrophizing is a mental or emotional overreaction to a certain incident, but it doesn't define your perspective of someone or something. Overgeneralizing is more potent as a cognitive distortion because it warps your entire sense of who you are, or of what another person or situation is, based on one isolated incident.

Emotional reasoning

This may be one of the clearest examples of cognitive distortion, and it is directly linked to our emotions. A common reason some people claim they hate love is that it makes you act stupid. In a way, it makes perfect sense what they mean; emotional reasoning is to blame here.

If a person has a romantic partner whom they are either infatuated or in love with, their judgment will likely be clouded. If this partner is not treating them properly, they are far more likely to excuse it due to their feelings—unlike their friends who probably want them to break it off. Their intense emotions and appreciation for this person make it hard to be truly objective about their actions.

The way this can become a cognitive distortion is through their reality becoming warped: Their partner may be bad for them, but they continue to stay with them, thinking it's worth it. When our emotions overpower our logic, it isn't always meaningful or romantic—sometimes, it can be damaging. The older we get, the better we tend to navigate these waters, but a good thing to do is to have an objective support system around you that can signal if you're ever succumbing to this emotional rationalization.

Fortune-telling

Not to be the bearer of bad news, but this one isn't as sweet as it sounds. We all wish we could sometimes definitively know the outcome of something without having to risk it first, but the fortune-telling we're talking about here doesn't let you do that.

I honestly believe that would be quite counterproductive. Knowing how our lives will turn out takes the accountability out of them, and therefore, the exploration. With this knowledge, we would stop trying altogether and simply let life happen *to* us, not *for* us.

Even if we aren't able to predict the future, some people's minds still attempt to—and, spoiler alert—they're not very good at it.

Fortune-telling in the form of negative thinking is what I lightly touched on in Chapter 1: We're not certain of what will happen, so we assume an undesirable outcome out of emotional protection. Does it emotionally protect us, though? Is thinking that we are bound to fail without even trying truly beneficial? Obviously, no.

Fortune-telling in a cycle of negativity only makes us do it again and again. To break out of it, we need to actively go against its nature. If your mind manages to convince you that you won't get that job—apply anyway! The only way to reprogram your mind is through conscious repetition. Just like my mother answering those anti-catastrophizing questions, it will eventually become second nature. Take chances, take risks, and stop letting your fortune-telling instincts influence you.

Mind-reading

Much like fortune-telling, this one is a bit of a guessing game. The same reasons we fortune-tell are behind mind-reading as well: We are too afraid of the unknown.

Mind-reading in the context of cognitive distortions boils down to assuming we know exactly what other people think and feel, especially what they think and feel about *us*.

When you aren't entirely sure what someone thinks of you (so, most of the time), you might be tempted to find out. When we like someone romantically, for example, many of us would pay good money to find out how they feel about us. Instead, we often resort to dissecting every little thing that they say or do. When we are left stumped and desperate for answers, we may start to create our own theories. When these theories get coupled with the anxiety or paranoia of not knowing, they tend to come out quite negatively.

This tendency to mind-read often leads us to feel worse about certain relationships than is necessary. If we managed to convince ourselves that someone doesn't like us, we might analyze every one of their actions as passive-aggressive, for example. Since most of us are not truly clairvoyant, our mind-reading attempts can be quite detrimental to ourselves and our relationships with others.

Imperatives

One of my favorite songs of all time is Beverley Knight's "Shoulda Woulda Coulda," though it's the kind of song I take in without paying much attention to the words. When you listen to the lyrics, however, Beverley sings about a deteriorated relationship and how her "shoulda woulda couldas" (her reflections on how things could have gone down) indicate that she is out of time. I don't believe in this; there is always time, at least to try again, if nothing else.

This song happens to showcase an instance of imperatives in terms of cognitive distortion. Imperatives occur when we make ourselves feel bad for feeling bad. If you have horrible anxiety when it comes to public speaking, for example, imperative thinking would cause you to think that you shouldn't have this anxiety. This thought process makes you angrier, more defensive, and less likely to be able to fix the issue. Only through acceptance of your anxiety can you go about making adjustments.

Inability to be wrong

Let's all admit it—it feels selfishly good to be right! It's that annoying little feeling that might overpower all others. In extreme cases, the inability to be wrong becomes a cognitive distortion.

When this is pushed to the extreme, the inability to be wrong makes a person prioritize being right over their relationship with the person they're arguing against, as well as over logic and proof. When someone fails to accept their errors, they not only put themselves against an impossible standard, but they risk losing the ability to learn from others. If you never see yourself as being incorrect about anything in the first place, then there isn't much room for that growth to occur.

Jumping to conclusions

This is a kind of distorted thinking that goes hand in hand with the inability to be proven wrong, fortune-telling, and mind-reading. Some of us are more guilty of this than others, and it's sometimes due to anxiety. If we have an anxious attachment style, for example, we may have the tendency to assume the worst of our partners. Imagine they had gone out to dinner with friends and hadn't texted you in three hours. Do you assume their phone is dead? Or maybe, they lost it? Or do you assume they got intoxicated and are now cheating on you?

Even without knowing the real answer, you may be so distraught at the thought of them betraying you that your whole night is ruined. The reality may be completely different than what we push ourselves to assume—jumping to conclusions is helping no one.

Labeling

We are constantly attributing labels to people, places, things, situations, and even ourselves. If we believe a certain family function is going to be awkward, then we don't attend; if we perceive someone at work to be 'fake,' we try to stay away from them; if we think of ourselves as a bad friend, we are more likely to act like one.

People with mental health problems or even self-esteem issues tend to put the most negative labels on themselves, and we all know how we can be our own harshest critics. If someone sees themselves as dumb, unattractive, or bad at their job, they eventually grow into that mold because their negative perception strips them of the will to work around those self-inflicted labels.

These labels focus on one aspect of a situation and discredit the others. By labeling, we are effectively throwing away potential and giving up on improvement.

Mental filtering

Just like a strainer, our minds will sometimes only remember certain parts of our past, whether it is consciously or not. Mental filtering is when a person only remembers the negative aspects of something. Perhaps you hated your time in high school, but why? Is it truly because everything was awful or do you simply happen to remember the worst of it?

We often say we hated a time in our lives because of something in particular that we didn't enjoy back then. However, by doing this, we diminish everything that we *did* enjoy. Maybe your last job was boring you out of your mind, but what if you really liked your coworkers? Does that period still hold an awful place in your past or could you acknowledge both the good and bad?

Minimizing

I think of minimizing as a present version of mental filtering: Rather than see the world for what it is (good and bad), a person focuses mostly on the bad. By minimizing our good experiences—no matter how small they are—we prevent our own experience of happiness. For example, when you chalk up your accomplishments to mere luck, disregarding the work you had to put into them, or when you acknowledge said work but tell yourself it was very easy to do, the victory doesn't count.

To stop minimizing, we need to actively fight against it. When you get the urge to think that something discredits your experience, try reframing your thinking to a more accurate representation of it.

Personalization

Personalization, or self-blame, happens when you take problems or details that have nothing to do with you and make them all about you. The textbook example is, of course, a child blaming themselves for their parent's divorce. Terrible, isn't it? As if we didn't already struggle enough with the things that directly pertain to us, we also carry the burden of guilt over things we have no control over. But that's exactly how overthinking and negative thinking in general work: They create a vicious cycle that's hard to break out of, spreading to include the things that should be peripheral to them.

Polarization

We've sort of been conditioned to see things in clear-cut spectrums; black or white, good or bad, yes or no, and so on. This is what we call polarization, or dichotomous thinking. This all-or-nothing state of mind makes it hard to approach issues with any nuance or room for compromise. But issues are complex, and shouldn't be boxed into one simple category.

In some cases, this can manifest as extreme indecisiveness. If you have two options to choose from and you are someone who polarizes their issues, you may be convinced that one of the options is right while the other is wrong. The pressure of wanting to choose the 'right' one is what makes it so difficult. In reality, however, both choices are probably fine but lead to different outcomes.

Another common example has to do with competitiveness. In this case, the person would be completely dissatisfied unless they felt like they were the best at something. This 'all-or-nothing' makes people feel inadequate and dissatisfied with something that they could still have considered an accomplishment.

Control fallacies

There are two ways in which control fallacies can manifest: The first comes when you feel desperate because you have no control over anything in your life and are therefore powerless to stop it; the second happens when you conclude that you have absolute control, and are therefore entirely to blame for any faux-pas.

Many people I know who suffer from control fallacies often oscillate between the two, and that's no way to live life. The ones that managed to escape this torturous mindset did so by consciously going against these trends. When they told me about how their life seemed to be spinning out of control, we worked together to find things that they felt like they *could* control. When the opposite happened and they were blaming themselves for every little thing going wrong, I helped them be at peace with letting go. Suffering through control fallacies can feel extremely isolating. Talking these feelings through with a trusted person may make you realize things aren't as dire as they seem.

Fairness fallacies

Life isn't fair, right? We've all heard this or said it ourselves a million times. But analyzing situations in terms of how just or unjust they are, not only falls under the dichotomous spectrum we've already discussed, but it also tends to be less than helpful in the context of mental health. This is especially true when we consider that fairness is not an objective thing, and will therefore change according to the person—what is fair to you might not be fair to the next person.

If someone in your life seems to be progressing faster than you are, your sense of envy might make you believe it's only their luck. Furthermore, why don't *you* have the same luck? It must be just an unfair distribution of luck, right? By believing this, you blame abstract factors rather than taking responsibility for your own experience.

Let's say your coworker got a promotion you were trying to get—do you think this is unfair? If you do, you are more likely to stay focused on this one failure rather than thinking of ways to improve your future.

Change fallacies

Believing that someone or something will eventually change to suit your needs is a fallacy of change. When I had my first serious boyfriend at 19, I constantly believed things would get better between us if he just grew up a bit more. It boiled down to me projecting my own needs and desires onto him and then getting disappointed when I didn't see the results I expected. He was certainly no angel, but I do take responsibility for the fact that I hadn't ended it sooner—I *chose* to stay and wait for him to make the changes; I could have reacted accordingly and cut him loose the moment I picked up on that, but I kept hoping he would change. More often than not, if someone is not willing to meet your needs, the only thing that needs to be changed is your approach.

Untangling Cognitive Distortions

Now, not every pattern of negative thinking will fit neatly into one of the definitions listed in this chapter, and they can even overlap. You probably related to most of these examples, remembering one time or another where you were guilty of them; I relate to some of them more than others. What usually happens is that one case of negative thinking leads directly to another, then another, creating a complex chain that is hard to break. Thankfully, by doing the necessary work, you can get there. It all starts with recognizing if any of these negative thinking types are recurring in your everyday life, on the brink of forming a habit, if you don't already have one. Once you've identified problem areas, there are ways to fight back.

Key Points

Let's look over the most important takeaways from Chapter 3:

- There are 16 types of common negative thinking
- It's important to understand and assess our symptoms of negative thinking in order for us to make the necessary changes

- We often get so used to these types of negative thinking to the point where we don't realize that we are not being objective
- Admitting our negative thinking tendencies is the first step toward improving our positivity

Chapter 4
Negative Thoughts: How and Why They Occur

"What we think determines what happens to us, so if we want to change our lives, we need to stretch our minds."

— *Wayne W. Dyer*

I'm sure I'm not the first to tell you that the brain remains a major mystery of ours, and the parts of it that we do understand are very complex. If you aren't the most technical person (such as myself), you won't want to learn every intricate detail of negative thinking on a neurological level. I am a strong believer, though, that knowing some basics of how our brains function allows our experiences to not only be validated but seem less abstract. Negative thinking has very real, biological explanations that help us understand why it occurs and how we can deal with it.

Stressing About Stressing

Constant stress is bad for you—we're all aware of this, but do most of us even know why? Beyond just the unpleasant feeling of being under constant pressure, the issue lies deeper.

The amygdala in our brains is a small, almond-shaped part of our brain that is largely responsible for emotional management, as well as processing threatening stimulants. However, its respective size and the strength of its connections with the other regions within the brain determine how strongly a person reacts to such stimuli. For example, a study at the Stanford University School of Medicine found that the larger a child's amygdala and the stronger its connections were, the more anxiety they experienced in everyday life (Bergeron, 2013).

What, you may ask, causes the increase in size of the amygdala? Several things, unfortunately, including anxiety and depression; but, among that list is a factor common to most of the population: stress. Chronic and heavy stress not only shrinks the prefrontal cortex of the brain (which could affect a person's social behavior), but it simultaneously enlarges the amygdala. This, in turn, makes a person's brain far too receptive to stress, meaning they can become overwhelmed from much less.

Cortisol

To put it simply, our stress causes the production of cortisol. Whenever we are stressed or under pressure, our brain triggers the production of this specific hormone that influences us in several ways. Cortisol is produced and released in the adrenal glands, which are little, triangle-shaped parts located atop each of our kidneys; these are our body's main stress hormones—our built-in alarm system. If danger strikes, cortisol kicks in and we are locked into fight-or-flight mode.

You might be thinking "A-ha! So cortisol is to blame for me being so anxious all the time." The truth is, cortisol is an integral part of being human and has helped our species to survive for as long as we have. Not only has it been helpful in life-threatening situations where time was of the essence, but it is also responsible for:

- Regulating your blood pressure
- Controlling your sleep cycle
- Keeping various inflammation down
- Increasing your blood sugar
- Managing the carbohydrates, fats, and proteins you consume
- Boosting your energy levels

With a list of such benefits, it's hard to believe that something so helpful can also be quite damaging. Let's put it this way: Imagine cortisol is an employee and your body is the company it works for. That employee is a valued member of the company, providing great work within reason and delivering great results. But the moment that employee is overworked and pushed around by the company, their productivity is hindered and they can no longer provide the ideal results, through no fault of their own. In the case of cortisol, then, if your body keeps perceiving danger and setting it in motion, the hormone's production will be sent into overdrive. Before long, the little tasks that cortisol performs, which were listed above, are thrown out of whack and start being threats themselves.

Your needs differ at different times; this is especially relevant in the case of perceived danger. If your body is on high alert, for example, cortisol can alter or shut down functions that get in its way, such as your digestive, reproductive, and immune systems. After the danger or pressure has subsided, your cortisol levels should calm down, meaning your bodily functions should be brought back to normal. If you're under constant stress, however, the alarm button stays on, causing your body's most important functions to potentially derail, leading to several health problems, including:

- Chronic headaches
- Heart disease
- Memory and concentration problems
- Digestion issues
- Trouble sleeping

- Weight gain
- Anxiety, depression, and other mental health issues

Now, do keep in mind that there are certain medical conditions that can produce too much cortisol, such as having a nodule or mass in your adrenal gland, or a tumor in your brain's pituitary gland. Too much cortisol can cause the condition known as Cushing's syndrome, leading to rapid weight gain, easily-bruised skin, muscle weakness, diabetes, and other health problems. Cortisol in low volumes, on the other hand, can lead to Addison's disease, which results in fatigue, diarrhea, and other issues.

Under normal circumstances, however, what keeps people under stress (therefore, producing more cortisol) is their own perception of the world. If their brains are wired to perceive everything unknown as a danger, then the body responds accordingly by creating more and more cortisol, possibly causing the whole system to go haywire.

The big takeaway here is that negative thinking is a much-needed reaction for our bodies due to the benefits of cortisol. This is exactly why I take so much issue with people wanting to eradicate negative thinking; that is not only unnatural and impossible, it's simply illogical. We need our negative impulses to navigate this rocky world around us, otherwise we *would* fall victim to its dangers. Issues only arise when we start seeing danger when there is probably none—we become a danger to ourselves. We need to reframe those negative thoughts and adapt to them, not get rid of them.

Brain Fog

Chronic stress is also a very common cause of brain fog—a state in which a person feels particularly forgetful, unconcentrated, and has a lack of clarity. Brain fog is often coupled with feeling physically tired, but not always; it has many different potential causes, ranging from pregnancy to various physical illnesses.

Another cause of brain fog happens to be the high production of the previously mentioned hormone of cortisol. Too much of this stress hormone tends to overwhelm the brain, exhausting it to the point of its inability to properly function. This affects nearly every region of the brain in a similar way to how chronic lack of sleep does—all of our mental functions start to suffer.

Brain fog can last continuously for several months if your brain is extremely overwhelmed or if no adjustments are occurring. If a person is not aware of what brain fog is or places a rigid amount of pressure on themselves, they might not even know they are experiencing it or will force themselves to simply push past it. Unfortunately, both lead to negative outcomes that only worsen the symptoms. They might start forgetting more and more deadlines, making errors in their work even with proofreading, and having their overall productivity and well-being suffer.

The only truly effective solution to brain fog is to stop doing what you're doing. What I mean by this is that your life requires a complete overhaul if your brain fog has been consistently getting worse or has lasted for more than a week. In this scenario, de-stressing isn't just an option, it's imperative.

Mental Health Complications

Negative thinking has many potential sources. We've gone over how time period trends, societal standards, and cultural differences can influence us to think one way or another. There are more reasons, however, that take control away from us.

No one asks to be mentally ill or go through traumatic experiences, yet they continue to happen to people. They might blame genetics, family members, or simply chance, depending on what caused them to have this fate. Understanding what other factors might influence your negative thinking can help you find the appropriate route to recovery.

Chronic negative thinking is a common result and symptom of PTSD, or Post-Traumatic Stress Disorder. PTSD is a mental health issue that follows a traumatic or particularly distressing event. A lot of people associate this illness with something like military combat, but in reality, PTSD can arise from an array of different experiences.

Even without PTSD, a person's rough history can influence their mental health to become significantly more negative. Experiencing emotional abuse growing up or having emotionally absent guardians can cause the child's brain to develop in a way that makes them more susceptible to depression, anxiety, attachment issues, and consequently, negative thinking.

Importance of Sleep

It is considerably easier to treat problems and fix issues when we can *see* them—at least, in a way that makes it undeniably clear that they are indeed real. With issues that have effects on our mental well-being, many of us struggle to understand what has to be done.

When someone breaks their arm, the protocol is clear: get to a hospital, get a cast put on, wait six or so weeks for it to somewhat heal, and take off the cast. You don't wait six months before going to the hospital, hoping it heals on its own, and you certainly don't go back to using your broken arm after putting a mere band aid on it. So, why do we do this so often to our mental issues?

The science is quite clear on the fact that our physical health influences the health of our brains, their functioning, and their mental well-being. Even if we do not physically see a concrete connection between the two, it is unquestionably there.

Sleep Is for the Strong

The effects of chronic lack of sleep on your mind include:

- **Lower alertness and concentration.** Sleep is a critical time for the brain. It's vital for the brain's plasticity, memory consolidation, and simply giving it a rest from conscious thought and focus. Without this rest, the brain cannot hold attention for nearly as long as it could otherwise and can't react as adequately to stimuli. The brain is like a muscle—if you keep working it out without any rest, it will eventually fail to pick up the dumbbell.

- **Worsened memory.** The REM (Rapid Eye Movement) cycle of sleep is a time for the brain to build and strengthen the memories it has created throughout the day. If this stage of sleep is not reached or is of poor quality or short length, the brain fails to adequately do so. Not only does it retain much less information, but in some cases, it can even create *false* memories.

- **Lack of cognitive flexibility.** If the brain is exhausted, running on extra time, it cannot possibly adapt to an array of new things. With proper sleep and good cognitive flexibility, a person's brain can easily adapt to a new environment or situation. However, without those factors, the brain is incapable of handling such new information and figuring out how to act accordingly. This makes meeting new people, starting a new job, and even hearing surprising news difficult to handle.

- **Worse emotional processing.** With a lack of sleep, your brain's efficiency is suffering. This is true even on a one-time basis; if you were to pull an all-nighter just once, the following day you are instantly more likely to be in a bad mood, react strongly to minor inconveniences, and manage your emotions poorly. If this occurs even from one night, imagine how it would look on a near-daily basis. Basically, negative thinking skyrockets as a result of poor sleep.

- **Poor decision-making.** Ever feel indecisive due to negativity? Well, this is multiplied if you're a victim of a rough sleep schedule. Without the proper seven to nine hours of sleep, your brain is running on overdrive, not knowing which way is up. With your brain being less capable of fully grasping the stimuli it's being presented with, it has a harder time understanding what the best response would be. If you're forced to make tough decisions, not only will this seem even more stressful than usual, it will feel riskier, as well.

There are several recommendations to get your sleep schedule on track. We've all heard them, but only a few of us actually follow through. I'll present a few tips that helped me straighten out my sleep schedule after a few years at an extremely demanding job, which are now simply part of my habitual routine:

- **Have a bedtime!** I used to be the type of person to go to bed when I felt really tired and not a minute earlier. There's a reason I did this, which is common to many of us: revenge bedtime procrastination—the act of going to bed later in favor of doing things you didn't get to do throughout the day. Oftentimes, the tasks that we end up doing instead of sleeping are hobbies or methods of relaxation that we simply do not have time for during the daytime. If you finish work late, you might be eager to get an episode of your favorite show in before you go to sleep. The victim in this scenario still ends up being yourself—or rather, future-you waking up the following morning. Another thing to look out for is something called the "second wind." This is a term used to describe a sudden increase in energy levels after you had been feeling tired in the evening. This second wind often fools people into thinking they shouldn't go to bed when really it is the body's last resort to try and help you do the things you're staying up for. Once I realized that it was merely my second wind giving me the ability to stay up until 1:30 am, I started listening to my body for the first time.
- **Kill the blue light.** Ah, yet another flaw of technological progress—the blue light. The blue light wavelengths emitted by various technological devices, such as your phone, laptop, and TV are all damaging your body's natural circadian rhythm. Now, we might not be able to avoid it completely, but there are ways that you can lessen the harm it causes you. Buying blue light glasses is one great way, but the best I can recommend is to simply put away your devices at least one hour to half an hour before bed. If this goes against your habits, it might be tough to kick, so try finding an equally-engaging replacement;

this could include an adult coloring book, doing some light bedtime yoga or stretching, reading a pleasant book, or going for a calming walk. I'm someone who gets bored easily, so I tend to rotate between these options; I was shocked at how nice it was to look at something other than my phone screen right before bed.

- **Treat your wind-down routine as non-negotiable.** Arianna Huffington—businesswoman and founder of *The Huffington Post*—is a very prominent advocate for the importance of sleep. She says that "a set ritual helps tell your mind and body that it's time to begin to wind down. My own involves turning off all my electronic devices [...] Then, I take a hot bath [...] Sometimes I'll have a cup of chamomile or lavender tea" (Kondo, n.d). If someone as busy and impressively successful as Arianna Huffington can make a relaxing wind-down routine a priority, it should inspire others to do so as well. She has a great point: Our bodies get used to habits and start to recognize triggers. If you incorporate a relaxing routine at nighttime, eventually you will not only crave it, but you will likely fall asleep easier.

Key Points

Let's look over the most important takeaways from Chapter 4:

- The effects of negative thinking go beyond just a bad mood
- Continuous negative thinking can cause some physical symptoms and make life even harder to live
- Aspects such as sleep and physical health should not be overlooked when trying to improve our negative thinking— they play a very large role
- Over-productivity and lack of rest ultimately lead to worse productivity

Chapter 5
A Skewed Perception

"Chains of habit are too light to be felt until they are too heavy to be broken."

— *Warren Buffet*

As rational as we may think we are, people are extremely biased—we often fail to be objective. Like many other psychological phenomena, this may come from both environmental and innate factors.

Briefly mentioned in Chapter 1 was impact bias—the phenomenon responsible for us overestimating our potential happiness and potential sadness. According to a study by Timothy Wilson and Daniel Gilbert (2005), one of the biggest contributors to our impact bias is focalism. Focalism is kind of like tunnel vision; when we imagine something awful happening to us, such as a painful breakup for example, focalism causes us to focus solely on this event. Realistically, if you were to break up with your romantic partner, that would not be the only thing happening in your life. At first, it may feel like it is, but quite soon the realization will start to set in that you have dozens of other things going for you. Focalism, however, makes us forget the influence of those other events in our life, even throughout a drastic event.

Another thing to remember is that people are constantly bored. We are built to be constantly craving something more, something new. How is this relevant to impact bias? Well, if impact bias causes us to expect ourselves to become considerably happier once we finally get that promotion we've wanted, it will not be enough. Why? Because we will get bored.

Boredom facilitates change (or, at least, it should). People are meant to get so used to their circumstances that they get bored and start to think innovatively to improve them. Therefore, when you finally get that long-awaited promotion, you *will* be happy, but not for nearly as long as you may have thought. Instead, you will get accustomed to this new life of yours and will soon enough have your eye set on something even bigger. Now, the same is applied to unpleasant future situations as well. You may be completely heartbroken for a few weeks, months, or even a year following your breakup, but you *will* eventually get bored of that as well. You are made to get used to your circumstances—good or bad. No feeling will remain constant throughout your life; you will likely want new things, no matter how many you get.

Negativity Bias

It's a known fact that we tend to dwell on the negatives much more than we do on the positives. Of course, the severity of this varies from person to person, but most people need to make an active effort to balance out what they focus on. Choosing to dwell on the positives requires a conscious decision for change.

Criticism has a greater impact than praise, just as bad news draws more attention than good news—it's no wonder you see nothing but tragedy every time you turn on your TV. You'll rarely see headlines about major positive changes around the world, but something negative will loom on almost every page of the newspaper. Partly, this is because paying attention to something negative can literally save someone's life, whereas noticing something positive simply boosts our moods. Another reason for this is that negative events have a greater impact on our brains, which some psychologists refer to as "the negative bias" (or negativity bias). This bias can have a powerful effect on your decisions, behavior, and even your relationships.

The negativity bias is your tendency to not only register negative stimuli more easily but also to overwhelmingly dwell on those triggering events. It's a psychological phenomenon that explains, for example, why bad first impressions are so difficult to overcome, or why traumas of the past tend to have such long, lingering effects. In pretty much every interaction we have, we are more likely to both notice and remember the person's negative aspects far more than the positive ones. You could be having the best day ever, receive some disappointing news, and have that be enough to ruin your otherwise perfect day. Essentially, your bias makes you pay much more attention to the bad things, giving them far more significance than they have. Negativity bias effectively causes us to turn over our emotional control to unpleasant events.

The negativity bias starts to emerge in infancy. Babies tend to pay greater attention to positive facial expressions and tones of voice, but this all changes when they reach one year of age. Around this stage, and sometimes earlier, babies begin to experience greater brain responses to negative stimuli. This further tips us off that the negativity bias is indeed more innate than it is cultivated through our worldly experiences.

Neuroscientific evidence shows us that there is a greater process of response in the brain to negative stimuli, even in adulthood. Psychologist John Cacioppo performed a test by showing participants several pictures of either positive, negative, or neutral scenarios; he then observed the electrical activity in the participants' brains and found that the negative images produced a much stronger response in the cerebral cortex than either of the other two categories of pictures (MIUC, 2017). Several factors have been identified so far as being responsible for our negativity bias.

Motivation

Research suggests that the negativity bias influences one's motivation to complete any task. Much like how some people thrive under pressure, we tend to have less motivation when there is something to be gained from our work than when there is something to be lost. Silly, isn't it? This means that if your boss promises you a bonus for meeting a certain quota, you'll be less motivated to meet it than you would be if you were threatened with being fired instead. The reason for this is that we are so wired to focus on the negatives that even if you are promised something good, like that bonus, you will still be more focused on what you might lose in the meantime (for example, hours of rest). If you were instead threatened with being let go, then you already know what you stand to lose. This is not a push for toxic work environments or draconian methods of leadership, but rather an explanation of how powerful our fear is.

Bad news

If you diligently check the news on the daily, you are likely to meet with tragedy after tragedy. This is because media outlets picked up on the negativity bias a long time ago and choose to exploit it for views and popularity. Pain, gruesomeness, and disaster have a shock factor—or wow factor—that allows that type of news to gain a lot of traction, quickly. The negativity bias also causes us to believe bad news over good news, much like how we believe an insult to be true much more easily than a compliment.

With this constant influx of negativity from the news, we are further programmed to receive it more easily. This, in turn, causes us to be more susceptible to it from other sources as well, and even expect the worst for our future selves.

Politics

In a world as politically unstable as the one we currently live in, generalizations are often hard to make. People that make up a certain political party may often be lumped into a stereotype by opposing parties, but in reality, tend to have some differing beliefs. Regardless, statistics offer us a perspective of trends that we may choose to deduce information from or not.

So far, psychologists have found that conservatives tend to have stronger responses to negative information than liberals do (Gjersoe, 2017). People who consider themselves politically conservative are more likely to rate ambiguous stimuli as threatening, causing opposing party members to view them as rather defensive in regard to hot-button topics. These differences might explain why some people are more likely to value things such as tradition and safety, while others are more in favor of rapid change and progress.

Suffering the Consequences

All of the listed factors above can help us understand the source of our negativity bias and why it is so potent in our lives. The following section will focus on the *outcomes* of negativity bias and why it can be quite harmful.

Relationships

The negativity bias can have a profound effect on your relationships; particularly, it can lead to you expecting the worst from others, even without having any real supporting evidence for this assumption. You might expect your parents to react badly to a decision you've made, such as a career change. If your defense system is already on high alert, chances are that the moment one of your parents says something as innocuous as, "are you sure?", you may perceive it as confirmation of your negative suspicions. Overall, our negativity bias makes us eager to confirm our negative expectations.

Where relationships are concerned, it's important to remember that negative comments carry more weight than positive ones; and since everyone is predisposed to a negativity bias, being aware of your tendency to fixate on the negative, you can start finding ways to let others off the hook a bit more.

Decision-making

Nobel Prize-winning researchers and friends, Kahneman and Tversky, once found that when making decisions, people often place greater weight on negative aspects than they do on positive ones (Lewis, 2016). This tendency is bound to have an impact on the choices people make and the risks they are willing to take. Going back to the career change example, maybe you want to switch lanes for all the best reasons: your current job isn't fulfilling enough, it doesn't pay as well as you'd like, and the people you work with are a bit toxic. Just as you start tossing the idea around of finding a new job, you start worrying about what might happen if you quit—that you won't make any income, that the employment gap might look bad on your resumé, or that you could wind up at another job that's just as bad, if not worse—and you ultimately decide against it.

Most of us go through life afraid of taking truly big chances because we believe we wouldn't be able to bear it if the results weren't positive. Big rewards come with big risks, no matter how inconvenient that may be. If we don't take the risk, then there are simply no results to reap of any kind, be they positive or negative. Assuming the worst possible outcome does not protect you from the bad, it only prevents you from getting the good.

People perception

To our caveman mind, the unknown equals danger. For this same reason, bad first impressions are *really* hard to shake off. When we do not know someone, we will make our conclusion based on the little information that we are provided with. If during our first meeting they happen to be 15 minutes late, that is all that we have to go off of, making us instantly perceive them as unpunctual and even perhaps disrespect-ful. The same approach can apply to settings and situations; if you have a bad experience somewhere the first time around, it's very likely you won't want to return to that place again.

Pining for Victimhood?

There is another possible psychological explanation for negativity bias. Except, not many people ever consider it and even fewer people will admit to it. The phenomenon I'm talking about is something I like to call "the weaponization of victimhood."

The term "underdog" is coined to represent someone who is perceived as less likely to succeed against their competition. Except, even the word itself has now gained certain respectability; people often tend to root for the underdog, not in spite of their proneness to failure, but *because* of it. This has rightfully given a certain power to people in positions of lesser authority than others. They are effectively uplifted by others' support to see them succeed against all odds.

In many societal issues, this is a fantastic thing to see—people who are the victims of injustices or mistreatment being supported and rooted for by others. However, this phenomenon can inspire some people to seek support *through* victimhood.

For example, a person may always blame their circumstances, other people, or pure chance, for all their misfortunes. Now, we have all had wrenches thrown into our lives seemingly out of the blue; however, if someone fails to take accountability for absolutely every mishap in their life, they are likely seeking pity for validation. They might want their life to seem harder and more unfair than everyone else's so that their short-comings are not blamed on them.

This mechanism of pining for victimhood not only takes away from the severity of real victims of injustice but makes negativity the default outlook of the individual themselves.

Snap Out of It!

If you feel the negative thoughts creeping in and you want to push your-self out of that situation, then the best thing to do is to immediately dive into something else altogether—something that you love doing and that is sure to keep your mind busy with positivity. Our mood greatly influences the way we think, as well as the other way around, so if you choose to do something satisfying, your mood will be uplifted and your thoughts will follow suit. If you start overthinking or spiraling into negativity at work, for example, then your options are not as broad as they otherwise would be. However, even doing something mundane can help take your mind off of negative thoughts, as long as you aim your focus at something else. So, at work, simply try giving it your all; boring or not, thoughts only have power if you give them attention. If you have a void in your positivity, fill it with accomplishments!

Establishing New Patterns

It's important to keep in mind that the solutions mentioned above might be quick fixes, but not long-lasting, let alone permanent ones. The entire premise of this book is to decrease excess negativity by turning it into something positive; but, before I get to explaining how to do so, we need to establish how one should go about *managing* their negativity.

Stop negative self-talk

If you start paying attention to the type of thoughts that run through your mind, you will probably be able to pick up on specific patterns. If you perhaps tend to think "I shouldn't have said what I said, I bet I offended them," pretty often, it may be indicating an underlying issue. This type of thought can mean any number of things: Maybe you need to start being mindful of people's feelings *before* you say something; or, perhaps you have some form of social anxiety that leads you to pick away at everything you say to others, even when no harm is done.

Reframing your habitual negative thoughts includes assessing them: Are they telling you something about yourself?

<u>Savor positive moments</u>

Since it takes more effort for us to recognize and remember positive experiences, making sure that you give extra importance to them when they happen can help you see the world in a more balanced, less nega-tively-biased way. Even if all it is, is being extra mindful of your morning coffee, it's worth doing—little tweaks can lead to the biggest changes. You do it so often that it's easy to disregard how much you enjoy it, but if you were suddenly stripped of that simple pleasure, you would miss it like crazy. You could even try replaying positive moments in your head the same way you do to the negative ones and think about all the good feelings they gave you.

Key Points

Let's look over the most important takeaways from Chapter 5:

- The negativity bias is ingrained in our brains, often making us notice the bad far more than the good
- The negativity bias affects every area of our lives
- Not taking accountability for our failures hurts us in the long run—playing the victim every time prevents us from growing
- Breaking out of the cycle of the negativity bias requires a change in habits and consistency

Chapter 6
Practical Steps Towards a Happier Life

"Happiness depends upon ourselves."

— Aristotle

A simple quote, isn't it? It's one of my favorites, and yet its significance doesn't click for us until we internalize its meaning.

Since negative thinking is going to be a part of us whether we want it to be or not, we might as well turn it into something productive. In this chapter, we explore how to use negative thoughts to your benefit, directly proving that getting *rid* of negative thoughts is not the solution to obtaining happiness—only reframing them is.

Ancient philosophers like Marcus Aurelius, Seneca, and Epictetus often practiced an exercise called *premeditatio malorum*—the "premeditation of evils." This activity aimed to foresee the negative things that could happen in life, such as losing one's job and becoming homeless, for example. Those philosophers believed that by imagining the worst-case scenario in advance, they might overcome their fears of negative experiences and therefore prepare for them ahead of time. So, while most people around them were focused on reaping success, those philosophers thought about how they might manage failure. That way of thinking is known as inversion and it can be a great skill to master.

Inversion

Inversion puts the focus on errors and setbacks which may not be obvious at first glance. It makes you assess an outcome you wouldn't want in a way that allows you to think through it rationally, and it starts by you asking yourself how *not* to do something. After all, sometimes it is far more important to consider why people fail at anything rather than how they succeed; success can be hard to emulate, but it's important to know what you can and should avoid. For example, if you're trying to think of innovative ways to get a work project to the next level, you can start by listing the things that would get in the way of it being finished or promoted. By identifying the most likely flaws and barriers that you might succumb to, you can become aware of how to remove, avoid, or prevent them. In addition, you might even be able to get some great ideas on what should be done just by doing the opposite of what you now know you *shouldn't* do.

This method of thinking falls in line perfectly with the notion we're now accustomed to: that people take in negative stimuli more readily than they do positive stimuli. Furthermore, it doesn't shame you for this tendency of yours, but rather, encourages you to use it to your benefit. So, if you think, "how can I alienate a customer?", you will know what not to do and, by default, what you *can* do to attract said customers. On the other hand, if you were to sit down and think, "how can I attract customers?", you're bound to have a harder time brainstorming ideas. Below are a few practical examples of inversion thinking you can apply to your day-to-day life, courtesy of best-selling author James Clear (n.d).

Project Management

Clear defends an application of inversion thinking dubbed "failure premortem." It starts with you taking into account the most important project you're working on right now. It then asks you to fast-forward six months into the future and assume the project has failed; how did that happen? What did you do wrong? So, essentially, it is asking you to think of your most important goal and to ask yourself, "what could make this possibly go wrong?"

This strategy is also known as the "kill the company" exercise because it can be used to spell out how a company might fail based on any given project. The key goal is to identify any potential challenges so that you can develop a plan to prevent them ahead of time.

It must be pointed out, however, that this should not become an obsessive or spiraling behavior. The entire point of project management inversion is being objective, without attaching any negative self-talk to the potential outcomes you're running through. To do so, you could use a few techniques; perhaps, try talking it out with a person who is impartial to the task. Another suggestion, if you are susceptible to negativity, would be to create a list of both possible failures and possible successes to balance out your perspective.

Productivity

Applying inversion thinking to productivity is my personal favorite. Procrastination is a massive problem for a large part of the population. We live in a world where we are constantly inundated with fresh new content coming at us from all sources, so it's easy to get distracted.

When you apply inversion thinking to your productivity, the question becomes, "what if I wanted to decrease my focus?" As in, thinking about how you can become distracted, rather than how you can avoid it. The answers to those questions will help you determine the interruptions that you should eliminate to free up your focus for what you have to do. If you know you're a sucker for a phone notification, try putting it on mute. If that doesn't work, start putting it in another room or in a place that is too inconvenient to access often. Once you've mastered the small things, you can broaden this approach by thinking bigger. For example, if you're aware that you procrastinate due to wanting to spend time with your friends, put your mind at ease by scheduling your meetups ahead of time. Thinking your distractions through before starting your work, leaves little room for spontaneous disturbances.

This insight reveals a principle that is important to remember, especially for those of us who tend to dwell on fears and negative thoughts: While chasing success blindly can have big consequences, preventing failure often carries very little risk.

Decluttering

The best-seller *The Life-Changing Magic of Tidying Up* by Marie Kondo applies inversion thinking to help people declutter their homes. The author's standout line is that "we should be choosing what we want to keep, not what we want to get rid of." In other words, your default setting should be to give up anything which does not kindle joy in your life. I put this philosophy to good use myself when I was sorting out my garage a few years ago. It is incredible, the number of things we keep around, gathering dust, just because we can't bring ourselves to discard them.

To apply this to your own life, stop going through your belongings during spring cleaning, looking for garbage to throw out. Instead, go in with the objective of finding what you truly treasure as a belonging. With this method, you may end up getting rid of a lot more junk than with the opposite approach.

Relationships

It's been known for quite some time now that nearly half of all marriages in the United States end in divorce (Wilkinson & Finkbeiner, 2022). I have a few theories on why modern marriages tend to dissolve so often, with most of them hinging on either personal or societal expectations. For now, though, let's brainstorm some possible relationship factors—what can bring about the end of a marriage? Is it a lack of trust? Of respect? Not spending enough time with one another or not having enough communication? Inverting a good marriage (or any relationship, really) can show you how to avoid a bad one. We often don't notice our faults until they are pointed out to us. To prevent frustrating your partner with your unforeseen imperfections, think ahead—could you be communicating with them better? Are you truly supporting them to the best of your abilities? This tactic of inversion simply shines a light on possible improvements before it's too late.

Personal Finance

Money: The cause of, and solution to, so many of life's problems. Debt accumulation, overspending, a lack of budgeting, and bad investments, are just a few factors that contribute to poor personal finances.

So, before you start worrying about how to earn more money, make sure you've figured out how not to lose it first. If you can manage to avoid that, you'll be ahead of most people, and ultimately save yourself a lot of anxiety. With personal finance, inversion thinking is pretty easy in theory: make an adequate budget; a budget that covers possible emergencies in addition to your wish list.

In conclusion, inversion thinking is a great way for you to reframe your negative thoughts, in order to apply them to something constructive. If your natural inkling is to always think of the worst-case scenario and stress about it, put your efforts toward finding solutions for it. Inversion thinking demonstrates perfectly why I was never supportive of stuffing down your negative thoughts in favor of artificial positive ones; instead, we have the capability of using negative thoughts to our ultimate benefit.

Personalized Solutions

Some people might wish that they could just take an antibiotic to rid themselves of pesky, negative thoughts. Unfortunately, there are no pills, supplements, or prescriptions that can cure your excessive negativity, like with a regular physical illness. Since the remedies are not as straightforward, each person is tasked with finding the best psychological solutions to fit their individual needs. What I mean, is that each of our brains functions uniquely and might require different approaches.

First, let's understand something called "neuroplasticity." Ultimately, the brain can change and adapt, proving that our thought processes, points of view, and habits are *not* set in stone. This fact directly contradicts people that say "oh, that's just the way I am," to explain a bad habit of theirs that they refuse to kick. In a way, yes, we do have some predetermined tendencies, however, they are never fixed. If there is something we want to change about the way we think, it's possible to do so more often than not.

There are two forms of neuroplasticity: functional plasticity and structural plasticity. The former corresponds to the brain's ability to reorganize its functions from a damaged part of the brain to a healthy one, while the latter is its ability to alter its physical structure.

What we'll be focusing on due to its relevance to this chapter, is called self-directed neuroplasticity. As the name indicates, this simply refers to when a person takes rewiring their brain into their own hands. How is this done? Often, through actively breaking a habit loop.

A habit loop is a cycle that explains why people partake in habits over and over again if they understand the damage it's causing them. Examples include checking your phone first thing in the morning, always stopping at a fast food drive-thru on your way home from work, leaving the dishes sitting in the sink to go do something else, etcetera. Why do we do all these things, knowing full well that they are hindering us? It's due to one vexing little habit loop composed of four parts:

1. **The cue.** The cue (also called the trigger) is what sets our habit loop into motion. It begins as soon as we notice a familiar environment, in which we tend to partake in a certain habit. For example, if you need to wash the dishes, your cue would be that you feel a sense of boredom rising up at the thought of actually doing it.
2. **The craving.** Once the cue is in motion, we instantly want to replace it with something more enjoyable. For the previous example, the sense of boredom from washing the dishes would make you instantly crave going to sit down on your couch and watch a show instead.

3. **The routine.** Following the call of the craving, we then partake in the habit that we've established by following through with what we truly want to do. You leave the dishes sitting in the sink once again and go to the couch. This is what leads to the fourth and last part of the habit loop.

4. **The reward.** Once we allow ourselves to partake in the habit, we are rewarded with feel-good hormones. This makes us feel satisfied for having followed our urges, rather than doing what we know is right. It is the release of these feel-good hormones that further reinforce our habits.

Notice-Shift-Rewire

The habit loop is directly related to the technique I'll describe in this sub-section. We now know that the feel-good hormones are so overpowering, that our brains lead us into making poor decisions over, and over, and over again. Habit loops are pretty much unavoidable if we don't take matters into our own hands.

The technique known as notice-shift-rewire is meant to help you break the habit loop of the negativity bias. Thankfully, it's a pretty straightforward process, but don't let its simplicity fool you—through dedication and repetition, it will get the job done, and your brain will mold itself to adapt to a new environment—one that doesn't allow it to default to excessive negativity. The following three steps make up this technique (Klemp, 2019):

1. **Take notice of the negativity bias**. This is perhaps the trickiest part to master, since we may be subjected to negativity bias so often that catching each instance is tough. This first step simply encourages you to be more mindful of your thoughts. If we experience rejection at work, for example, we need to bring attention to our thoughts if they mimic something like "I must not be good enough," or "my boss probably hates me." When these thoughts bombard your mind, take a second to reflect!

2. **Shift your mindset to something more positive: gratitude.** Once you've taken notice of your negativity bias, actively think of something that opposes it. If the automatic thought was "I must not be good enough," list what you are grateful for regarding yourself, your skills, and the job you have. You may even feel a small weight being lifted off your chest as you prevent yourself from spiraling. Gratitude is also known as one of the most powerful tools for creating new, better neural pathways.

3. **Rewire your brain!** Seems easier said than done, right? Well, this step gets its name from what it achieves *over time*. Meaning, it isn't a one-time fix, but it is easy enough for you to do it often; all you have to do is savor the good in your life. Take what you did in step two, and apply it on a broader scale, or just to remember good moments from the past—anything that gets you to notice the significance of the positives of your life over the negatives. Spend 15 to 30 seconds thinking of the positives and you will be one step closer to solidly rewiring your brain.

CBT Made Easy

Cognitive Behavioral Therapy (CBT) is a form of psychotherapy that is highly effective in improving one's overall life quality. It covers a wide range of issues, including depression, anxiety, eating disorders, relationship issues, substance use, and more. Generally, it is performed as talk therapy with a professional psychologist but has a high success rate when done solo as well. CBT done alone allows you to be your own therapist; you learn your triggers and become equipped to deal with many psychological and or emotional issues thrown your way.

The next time you feel your anxiety flaring up or your negative thoughts clouding your judgment, you can sit down and get ready to write. CBT suggests that you do the following:

1. Assess your level of distress. Pick a number range that makes the most sense to you, such as 1 to 10, 0 to 100, or what I tend

to choose for myself: 1 to 5. 1, for me, is a pretty relaxed state of being, while 5 indicates that I am actively being sucked into the void of negativity.

2. Next, make note of what had occurred to trigger this distress of yours. What thoughts automatically flooded your mind as soon as it happened? If you were set off by a low grade on an important exam, for example, think about what went through your mind as soon as you received the news. Was it, "I knew I would fail, why did I even try?" Or perhaps, "I am not made for this—I don't have the skillset"?

3. Think back to the categories of negative thinking presented in Chapter 3 and ask yourself if this reaction of yours exhibits one of the described types. Are you overgeneralizing by attaching too much importance to this one failure? Are you catastrophizing and feeling like your life is over because of this one fault? By knowing what type of negative thinking is occurring, you can begin to shift away from it.

4. Look for evidence that your emotional reaction to this trigger is not objective. If you are feeling like you don't have the skill set to ever pass this exam, what points to this being untrue? For example, you might have spent weeks preparing for this exam, proving that you *were* building up your knowledge for this exam; or, maybe you passed all the practice exams and were simply overcome with some nasty test anxiety that caused you to fail the official one.

5. Imagine you are a different person who is having a conversation with you about the situation. If you told your best friend that you are not intelligent enough to pass this exam, what would they say? If they're a good friend, they would most likely point out all of the reasons why you should not be feeling this way. Imagine what they would say—this forces you to take another perspective.

6. Using the previous steps, reconsider what happened, and reevaluate the severity of the situation without any cognitive distortions. You could ask yourself: Will this matter to me in

two years? Chances are, your negativity bias has temporarily made you forget about the rest of your life's successes.

7. Write down your thoughts and feelings on the event from a more objective standpoint, such as, "failing this exam made me feel disappointed, given how much time I spent preparing for it." The sentence shouldn't use any false positivity, but rather, just be an objective statement of your feelings.

8. Using the same scale as before, give a new score to how anxious, depressed, or otherwise distressed you feel.

CBT takes practice and commitment. Many people choose to start with doing this exercise several times per day before toning it down to less. Although CBT may seem like a short-term fix that applies to issues on a very individual basis, the repetition of it leads to the rewiring of your brain away from extreme negativity.

Key Points

Let's look over the most important takeaways from Chapter 6:

- Inversion thinking is kind of like applying reverse psychology to avoid negativity: it helps us take on another perspective and become more objective
- Inversion thinking can be applied to any area in which you feel like you struggle with overwhelming negativity
- Feeding into bad negative habits causes them to get stronger— if we do not make the effort to break them, we fail to move forward
- Notice-shift-rewire is a technique used to toss your brain out of a state of negativity, and with enough repetition, it may replace the habit of negativity
- CBT is a powerful form of self-therapy to provide a different perspective on a negatively-perceived situation

Chapter 7
Finding the Light at the End of the Tunnel

"Happiness is a direction, not a place."

— Sydney J. Harris

A lot of methods I will suggest for transforming your negative thinking don't have much to do with negativity at all. Instead, most of the heavy work will come directly from improving *other* areas of your life. A person who allows themselves to be happy and actively tries to enjoy their life is significantly less susceptible to being seized by negativity. For this chapter, I'll ask you to shift your focus to your life in general. We'll be exploring how strongly emotions intertwine with your outlook on life, changes you can make to improve your life's satisfaction, and the difference some simple lifestyle changes can make.

Emotions: Guilty or Innocent?

If you think back to the content in Chapter 2 regarding changes in mindset throughout history, you'll recall reading about the Romanticism era—a period full of art with subjective meaning and emotional expression. This was crucial in our development as a global society, as it was finally allowing us to focus on the value of immaterial aspects of life. This was precisely what psychologist Abraham Harold Maslow was exploring when he made the five-tiered pyramid called "Maslow's Hierarchy of Needs" (McLeod, 2020). This pyramid is meant to show what needs people focus on, according to the level of their necessity for survival and or life. For example, the bottom (and largest) section of the pyramid is physiological needs, such as food, water, and shelter. This means that these parts of life are the most essential for survival, and without them, most people wouldn't be focused on needs placed higher up on the pyramid. The top three tiers of the pyramid—belongingness and love, esteem, and self-actualization—are the ones that society had started to focus on, initiated during the Romanticism era. Unlike the bottom two tiers—physiological needs and safety needs—the top three are focused on emotional and mental elements. This goes to show that while we think of physical things as being essential for survival, attending to emotional needs is essential for *happiness*.

Now, to be clear, happiness will not erase your negative thinking, and nor should it. It does, however, prevent negative thinking from taking over your life.

So far, research has shown that the amygdala in happier people had the same level of activity when shown joyful images as it did when the individual was shown sad images (Allen & Smith, 2016). This alone is enough to indicate that happy people don't retain their positivity by ignoring the bad in their life, but simply that they attach an equal amount of importance to both the bad and the good. In happy people, the negativity bias is not triumphant—it is balanced out by how carefully they try to experience the good.

Making Time for What Counts

Time is in limited supply for us all. "Time is money," as Ben Franklin said (1748); but, I would argue that time isn't money—it's happiness.

We all dedicate time to what matters to us. To some, spending 60 hours per week at work satisfies their need to feel accomplished or wealthy; to others, spending a month traveling every year feels non-negotiable. Time is valuable because it's a limited resource that dictates how good we feel. Think of a day where nothing seems to be going right—your work took two more hours to complete than you expected, you were too tired to go to the event you were looking forward to, and you were too down in the dumps to do anything beyond binge watch a show. Chances are that the following day you might feel like the previous day was wasted since you didn't get to spend your time in a way that brought you joy. So, applying this to your everyday life, what should you do to avoid this feeling?

Time management is the answer, but it might not be what you are used to. When people are told to make a timetable for their day, many run to fill up their schedules to the brim, making productivity the goal. But should it be? What if the goal, instead, was satisfaction? This satisfaction does not have to be a surface-level guilty pleasure, but rather, it should include your work, your relaxation, and your progress. How much time do you need to spend on each of these to truly be satisfied with your day?

Burnout does not discriminate—it is the sense of extreme exhaustion, dullness, loss of passion, and even possibly depression. It creeps up on you bit by bit while you are out there, working passionately, thinking you are about to sprint to the finish line of success. Burnout is the unpleasant reminder that the journey to success should be treated like a marathon, instead. Being blinded by motivation or a passionate drive, we often lose sight of the fact that our time has to be divided more evenly. The true satisfaction of time management comes from this exact balance.

So, when I suggest that you time manage, I don't want you to go making a 30-point essential to-do list, working yourself to the bone. You should be dedicating your time to things you truly enjoy as well: spending time with loved ones, going outdoors, partaking in a hobby (no matter how silly), and overall, just taking time for yourself. This is a step to solidify your dedication to noticing the good.

A Shift in Mental Focus

When thinking of happiness, we need to remember one thing: we will always want more. There's a reason why most people think, "why don't billionaires just stop earning money?" Well, I can think of a few explanations, but the most accurate one is that they are not satisfied with what they already have. Crazy, right? Having 10 billion dollars only makes them want to make 10 billion more! To the average joe, 10 billion dollars is something we will never see, so to want 20 billion dollars seems simply ridiculous; and yet, this doesn't work in the psychology of a billionaire.

Humans have a very weird and confusing relationship between chasing after desires and feeling satisfied with achieving said desires. What we can get from this is key to understanding our journey toward happiness: it isn't a destination. A crucial thing to understand to be happy is that obtaining the things we desire is not enough in itself to make us happy —we have to find additional avenues.

Growing Your Self-Confidence

People walk a fine line when it comes to their relationship with themselves. On one end of the spectrum, they might be struggling to not see a failure in the mirror; on the other, they may feel like a God among men. Ego is something we all have, but not a lot of us understand exactly what it is or how to deal with it. Too much or too little of an ego is enough to ruin your life, just like the wrong amount of baking soda would do to a cake.

So, what is ego? Is it Narcissus, falling deeply in love with his reflection? Is it that irksome, guilt-filled satisfaction that arises when you realize you are doing better in life than those around you?

The word "ego" is Latin for the word "I," but it gets more complicated than that. In psychology, the concept of the human ego came into play when famous psychologist Sigmund Freud introduced it in the early 20th century. He explained it as a complicated part of ourselves that melds together our animalistic and moral tendencies, but nowadays, many people confuse ego with confidence. However, the difference becomes quite clear with a simple explanation.

Ego is when someone believes they deserve or will attain things simply because of who they are. Self-confidence, however, is believing they will attain things based on their objective merits, such as working hard for them. Compare the phrase, "I don't even have to try to get it," with the phrase, "I deserve to get it because I have been putting in the work." One exhibits a blind belief in yourself based solely on who you are, and the other is based on the conscious actions you made.

Self-esteem is kind of the best of both worlds from ego and self-confidence: It is how much we value ourselves, even if we are in a productivity slump. Low self-esteem often starts in childhood when you feel as if you are a disappointment to your loved ones or unable to meet their or your expectations. Self-esteem is further lowered when people are stuck in a negative mindset. Catastrophizing, overgeneralization, personalization, and minimizing all continuously contribute toward beating down your self-esteem. While these negative types of thinking continue, healthy self-esteem is extremely hard to achieve.

What you need to do to be happier is have a balanced ego, a healthy self-esteem, and lots of self-confidence. Easier said than done though, no? Well, luckily, there are several practical methods for you to try.

<u>Be kind to yourself</u>

If you've ever done some prior research on reframing negative thinking, I'm sure you've heard this one before. The difference is, I'll tell you precisely what I did to eventually achieve this colossal task. When I had stretches of difficult times in my 20s, I struggled a lot with my self-esteem. I tried many things, with very few results. It wasn't until I was completely fed up with feeling bad about myself that I took some radical steps.

First, I forced myself to be kind to myself—and I did this quite literally. Every morning, I would look in the mirror for one to two minutes straight, before coming up with at least five compliments to give myself.

Instead of choosing things I hated about myself and pretending like I liked them, I challenged myself to find aspects I truly felt good about. This made me discover that there *were* many things I liked about myself, but they got buried under the massive pile of my 'flaws.'

Within a few weeks of that exercise, I found a new objective for myself: to get comfortable with being uncomfortable. During that period of my life, I was a much smaller person—personality-wise. I felt truly myself when I wasn't worried about someone else's judgment. So, I decided to do things I perceived would make me feel embarrassed. For example, if I liked my outfit but was tempted to not wear it out of fear that others would think it looked bad, I wore that outfit. It was incredibly challenging at first and even emotionally tolling. However, when I would get home that night, I felt incredible; it made me realize that nothing *truly* bad happened just because I felt a little bit less conventional. Suddenly, the catastrophizing thoughts melted away; I eventually became unfazed by others' judgment—if they didn't like me, I no longer felt like I was an entirely bad person.

Practice being assertive

There are a lot of people who confuse assertiveness with a lack of tact. In my opinion, however, being honest with yourself and the other person is the most respectful thing you can do. If you are invited to an outing you know you don't want to go to, saying "no" does not necessarily mean you do not value them or their offer.

Assertiveness is an essential component of self-respect, and consequently, self-esteem. When we respect our time, our wishes, and our desires—all without sacrificing them to please others—we are inherently honoring our values. Saying "no" when needed is important to practice to increase your assertiveness, but it is not the only way. I would recommend thinking of it more as decreasing your passiveness, rather than increasing your assertiveness—at least, at first. If your coworker interrupts you with their idea, practice not being passive by speaking up and saying something like "excuse me, I'd appreciate it if I could just finish the point I was making." To someone who makes themselves smaller to appease others, this phrase might even seem rude or brash. In reality, it does not contain any disrespectful language.

Assertiveness also requires you to stop being constantly selfless. If you struggled to impress your family as a child, you might overcompensate now by doing the absolute most you can for everybody around you. To change this, treat your time as sacred. In the previous section of this chapter, we talked about prioritizing rest to prevent burnout. Now, we combine that with the notion that your time is yours, no matter how you choose to spend it.

Personally, I have a very firm rule: I will always make sure I have time to myself and will not sacrifice it for someone else unless I want to make that change or it is an emergency. If I made a firm plan to spend two hours working and one hour resting, I kindly say "no" to someone asking me to help them with something trivial during that particular time block. I value my time, my schedule, and the fact that I need both time to work and time to rest. Prioritizing your time is not selfish for you nor me—you cannot help someone when you yourself are struggling, so make your life the priority.

Setting boundaries

There's a reason that assertiveness was discussed above because you will certainly need to get comfortable with it to set boundaries. Setting boundaries is one of the most underrated and overlooked methods of ensuring healthy relationships; not just with romantic partners, but friendships, family members, and even coworkers. Due to them being often overlooked, many people don't even realize why some of their relationships are so draining.

Boundaries are an extremely personal thing. Some people have boundaries that we do not understand and vice versa. However, whether we understand them or not, they deserve respect. Oftentimes, someone establishing a boundary is a sign that they *want* to keep you in your life and not the opposite. So, think of boundaries as tools to ensure mutually respectful relationships.

Sometimes, people who drain us in one way or another are not of ill intent. Many of them may not even notice the effects of their actions. If someone is used to you saying "yes" to everything they ask of you, they will likely continue to unassumingly do so. For a time-draining relationship as such, you could establish a boundary by starting the conversation with something like, "I really value my own time, and from now on, I will only be available when my schedule and energy level allow it." If your counterpart reacts poorly to your boundaries, it is an indication that they profited from you not having any in the first place. The only relationships worth keeping are those where you both strive to be better for each other and respect each other's needs.

Key Points

Let's look over the most important takeaways from Chapter 7:

- As long as basic survival requirements are met, people achieve happiness through emotional fulfillment
- Time is a precious and limited resource—the things you spend time on are the ones that will be nourished the most
- People are meant to want more and more, failing to be satisfied with what we already have; don't assume you'll be happy forever once you achieve a certain milestone
- Self-confidence is required for true happiness and success— develop it by going outside of your comfort zone, being conscious of your thoughts, and don't be afraid to put yourself first

Chapter 8
Think Lovely Thoughts?

"Mindfulness isn't difficult. We just need to remember to do it."

— *Sharon Salzberg*

Positive thinking is so celebrated in mainstream media that it has become this sort of mantra for millions of people around the world. Everyone promotes it, from self-help gurus to Instagram influencers, and we all take it in as something we should be doing more of in our day-to-day. The problem is that positive thinking is generally said to operate by canceling out negative thoughts—which is something that's never going to work. Our negative thoughts will keep coming to us, and they don't deserve to be seen as this threat that needs to be vanquished. If we try to push them out instead of dealing with them accordingly, it would be the same as trying to push a plastic ball underwater—the moment we let go, it will shoot its way back to the surface. Besides, it's no help to tell yourself you don't feel a certain way when you do. My go-to example is always the finger cut: If you're in the kitchen and you cut yourself, then saying you're not wounded won't make the cut disappear, you still need to tend to it or there might be an infection, making things much worse.

In the context of positivity, trying to mask your negative thoughts can occur when you get the gut feeling that you don't like someone you've met. Say you're in a social setting and someone there is just giving you an icky vibe. Positive thinking essentially tells you not to humor those feelings and to instantly force yourself to like them, but it may very well be that your intuition is right and the person poses a threat to you. It would be of help to try and figure out why you feel something is wrong with that person. In reality, it could very well be that you simply don't like the way they are dressing or the number of tattoos they have, which might reveal some sort of inner prejudice within you that you could work on—it's always great when we recognize that there is room for growth within us! But maybe it will also make you watch your back, keep your belongings near you, and keep a close eye on the drinks you are served. Unless you have a direct problem with anxiety or paranoia, that icky feeling from the beginning may very well be saving you at times.

So, to sum it up, the key to handling negative thoughts is to acknowledge them, try to get to the root of why you are having them, and then react accordingly. In this chapter, I'll be introducing you to another key component of handling negative thoughts and preventing negativity bias: mindfulness.

How Mindfulness Fits Into Your Life

"Mindfulness" is a word that gets tossed around a lot nowadays. It gets tossed around not only by influencers trying to be relevant in the modern trend of caring for mental health but even by companies. Corporations and businesses have noticed this shift in mentality toward an emphasis on being present and mentally healthy. With this information, many of them have started to do something I like to call "mindfulness-washing" (originating from the idea of "green-washing"); they will pretend to be mindful to gain respect, attention, and new clients. This is quite literally the opposite of what mindfulness is meant for.

In the simplest of terms, mindfulness is about being present in the world around you. It originated in the Buddhist and Hindu religions that were briefly described in the second chapter. This ancient practice has no better time to be gaining popularity than right now, however. With so much of our lives revolving around money, social media, and technology, we often lose sight of what else we have around us. Even most jobs nowadays will have you staring at your computer screen for seven to eight hours a day. While you do this, the world still turns, the sun still shines, the wind still blows, and you might be forgetting about all of these pleasantries.

Mindfulness is a large component of Zen Buddhism—a branch of original Buddhism. Whether you are religious or spiritual in some capacity or not, mindfulness is a practice that goes beyond just its traditional objective of enlightenment. In today's world, it's used largely to give your brain a rest and to prevent burnout, since it slows your pace down.

The Effects of Mindfulness

Neuroscientist Zoran Josipovic believes that there are two networks in the brain: the extrinsic network and the intrinsic (default) network (Danzico, 2011). The former is responsible for focusing our attention on the external world, such as things we see or tasks we have to complete. The latter is in charge of focusing our attention on our internal world, such as thinking about ourselves and how we feel. However, these two networks are rarely equipped at the same time; instead, when one is really active, the other is barely functional. This would explain why people feel out of touch with themselves when they're stressed with work: their intrinsic network hasn't gotten to be active in a long time. Thankfully, mindfulness is supposed to provide us with a balance of the two.

In today's society, mindfulness is treated as optional; lots of people in the West don't see it as an important part of their lives. I didn't either, at first. We aren't exactly taught what mindfulness is in school or seminars, so I never heard about it until I was in my late 20s. To be honest, I didn't feel like it would make much of a difference in my thought process, but I tried it anyway because it seemed like a quick way to relax. I was both right and wrong; mindfulness does have an instant short-term effect on you in the form of relaxation, but it started to provide me with much more. I eventually started being mindful even when I didn't consciously make the choice to be. It became an ingrained habit that I easily applied to my entire life. Soon, I saw the most significant change it caused: I no longer felt as if life was zooming right past me—I started experiencing every day of my life. My days weren't a blur, my hours didn't pass me by, and I started to feel as if the things I spent my time and energy on were benefiting my journey.

I could go on and on about how important mindfulness is, but I'm sure the more useful approach to convince you of its significance is to present some proof. Well, scientific studies have shown that mindfulness has effects on several parts of the brain that span functions such as perception, complex thought processes, emotional management, introspection, pain tolerance, and sense of self (Congleton et al., 2016). At least four of those (complex thinking, emotional management, introspection, and sense of self) are highly beneficial to our cause of increasing positivity. When these four improve, we stop being as susceptible to anxiety, stress, and the negativity bias—all because our minds are stronger in resistance to negativity.

Another study was tasked with taking brain scans of people who meditate regularly. The researchers ended up scanning the brain of a Buddhist monk four times, with many years passing in between each scan. What they concluded from their last scan during which the monk was 41 years old, was that his brain appeared to have aged only 33 years —an entire eight years younger (Geggel, 2020). This acts as proof that things such as mindfulness, and therefore meditation, can physically improve the way our brains function.

Inhale, Exhale...

Mindfulness is all about acceptance, not change—similar to what I've been proposing throughout this book: don't *mask* your negative thoughts, *use* them. Accepting is all about opening up to your inner experiences, such as your thoughts and feelings. It involves an active and aware embrace of said experiences as they emerge, and allowing them to be present rather than attempting to change, minimize, or avoid them.

The most well-known approach to the practice of mindfulness and awareness is meditation. The core principle of all types of meditation boils down to accepting the external world and simply observing what you have going on inside. They generally start with you sitting or lying down, getting in touch with your body and your five senses, and then noticing your thoughts and emotions. With your eyes closed and your focus on your breath and body, the thoughts that are most important to you at that time will eventually pop up. Rather than getting frustrated that instead of ascending into some spiritual realm you are thinking about daily stresses, you let them be—you allow your mind to run its course. Anxiety is often caused by a whirlpool of emotions brought up by a thought, and the stronger we fight against it, the more violent it becomes. Meditation allows you to approach your mind as a neutral entity by allowing it to simply experience whatever it wants, without judgment.

Meditation is not the only approach to mindfulness, however. Although I am a big advocate of incorporating meditation into your everyday life, sometimes other techniques are better for beginners. The great thing about mindfulness is that ultimately, it is not an activity or an exercise—it is a lifestyle and a thought process; it may start as an exercise before spilling into every corner of your life. For this reason, I'd like to introduce a few non-meditative means of increasing your mindfulness.

Journaling

The first is journaling. Now, there is not just one way to journal—there are a limitless number of things that you can write. The type of journaling I'm referring to, however, is narrowed down to a few key points: getting in touch with your present self.

When I first started journaling, I would carry around a small journal almost everywhere I went. Whenever I felt overwhelmed, anxious, or any other unpleasant emotion, I would take it out and put all my thoughts down on paper. Nowadays, I've reduced my journaling to once per day, as soon as I wake up. If you are a morning person (or are trying to be) I recommend you do the same.

Keep a notebook and pen on your bedside table, and make this the centerpiece. When you first wake up, whatever you do, do not look at your phone. You might want to take five or so minutes to yourself, doing a mental run-through of your upcoming day, before reaching over and getting to some mindful work. If you want a structure, you could write down your thoughts or worries in bullet-point format and then provide a few phrases for each one, explaining why you feel that way. If you're like me and you prefer ultimate creative freedom, follow the 'stream of consciousness' technique. For this, the steps are very easy: Write down whatever you are thinking, no matter how much sense you think it might make or how pretty it looks. Allow your mind to throw itself onto the pages, making your feelings seem less than undefeatable. For some reason, seeing the way you feel written down in front of you can automatically make it seem more manageable.

Conversation

Who doesn't like spending a nice evening with the people whose company you enjoy the most? Hopefully not you, because for this next mindfulness technique, you'll need a casual conversation partner.

Just like journaling, there are not many rules here for you to follow. All I ask is that you listen to what the other person is saying while they are saying it. Easy, right? Well actually, many people don't realize how easy it is for us to think about ourselves even while we listen to others. More particularly, people tend to automatically start thinking of their response to what is being said to them before the person has even finished talking. On one hand, yes, you're prepared to continue the conversation. On the other hand, however, you may be failing to truly soak up the meaning of your conversational partner's words.

The next time you're talking to someone, focus all of your attention on them. What is their tone? Does their choice of words alter what they are saying? What is their body language like? Not only does this allow you to fully immerse yourself in the conversation from the other person's perspective, but you are solidifying your experience in the present moment—all that mindfulness is about.

Eating

"Mindful eating"—maybe you've heard of it, maybe you know someone who's tried it, but what is it exactly, and does it work?

The short answer is yes, it works. Mindful eating is a very easy concept to understand. What stops most people from using it is that it seems time-consuming. Ironic, though, isn't it? Anyone who wants to be more mindful of themselves and their thoughts should be trying to *escape* from the idea that everything has to happen as quickly as possible.

Mindful eating is similar to that of mindful conversation: You try to notice as much as possible. The twist, in this case, is that you must try to apply all your five senses.

Grab a bowl of food for your dinner and before consuming it all in front of the TV, try to do something different. First, take a look at it: How many colors can you count? Are there different shades of each color? What do you think the textures will feel like on your tongue? Then, apply your sense of smell; what are the smells you are experiencing? Does the smell remind you of anything? You can continue to ask similar questions as you go through every one of your five senses; is the plate of food hot to the touch? How many flavors can you taste? Does the food make any particular sound when you chew it or touch it with your utensil?

Many people go beyond their senses when doing mindful eating. In particular, they like to think about where the ingredients came from. As you take each bite, try to think of the origins of an ingredient in the food. Perhaps they originated halfway across the world, or maybe you grew it yourself in the backyard.

It is only through such laser focus that you can begin to honor your food, and therefore honor your relationship with it in the present moment.

Thinking Intentional Thoughts

Some people fail to realize the solid connection between mindfulness and negative thoughts. After all, what does the sound my food makes have anything to do with my anxiety? To answer that, we have to understand that every action we take, impacts our thought processes. This is not meant to scare you into over-analyzing everything you do or expect yourself to be perfect, but to think about the general trend of your actions. So yes, even paying attention to your meal or writing down your emotions once per day can end up making a large impact on how you view life, and therefore, the negativity bias.

Cognitive Defusion

This process complements your efforts to be mindful and to stop judging yourself for your thoughts and emotions; it requires you to take a step back, distance yourself from your thoughts, memories, and images, and objectively notice them as they are. This prevents you from attributing to them a label of any kind (such as "negative" or "painful").

There are three good ways to do this:

- "Just noticing": When you start having a negative thought, acknowledge it by saying, for example, "I notice I'm having the thought that I'm useless, again. That's the third time today."
- "Thanking the mind": When you take a moment to sarcastically give your mind appreciation for the unhelpful thought it ushered in, it helps you to realize just how silly the thought is, and that your original reaction to it was even sillier; this, effectively, takes away its power. "Ah, thanks a lot, brain, for making me feel useless for the third time today."
- "Repeating a thought": Interestingly enough, repeating a negative thought over and over again might make you realize that you have no reason to listen to it. If you repeat your thought out loud, especially if you do it in a funny voice or even by singing it, it will help you create more distance from it.

Key Points

Let's look over the most important takeaways from Chapter 8:

- You cannot treat negativity as if it does not exist—don't shy away from acknowledging your tendencies
- Our relationship with the present moment is key in preventing the negativity bias from taking over
- Mindfulness is the practice of solidifying yourself in the present moment and treating what goes on in your mind as neutral
- Mindfulness can and should be applied to many areas of your life—meditation is a great technique for mindfulness, but it is not the only one
- The concept of cognitive defusion allows us to disconnect from our pesky, negative thoughts through three different possible techniques

Chapter 9
Seeking Motivation

"You are never too old to set another goal or to dream a new dream."

— *C.S Lewis*

Negativity can zap everything enjoyable about life right out of it. Your passions, your interests, your hopes, your dreams, and your curiosity, to name a few. Another key component of life that falls victim to ravenous negativity, is motivation.

Motivation is the bread and butter of our enjoyment of life. It differs for each of us and steers us into individual paths, but without it, life can become quite dull; projects that you used to look forward to no longer seem interesting; the hobbies you wanted to try pursuing have transformed into simple time-wasters that you don't see the point for. When things that are meant to give you an interest in life are lost, you may become disappointed in yourself. Losing your motivation can become a very slippery slope to an unsatisfactory life or even, possibly, depression.

Excited, Not Afraid

There are two types of people in the world: those who are intimidated by unpredictability and those who are inspired by it. Neither group is wrong, since unpredictability can exhibit both factors; however, one group is certainly being a little held back by their perspective.

I always say that the most predictable thing about life is that it will always be unpredictable. We can always count on it to throw in surprises that we are expected to deal with (both good and bad). The way we feel in anticipation of these surprises can either set us up for success or failure. Your negative thoughts and the way you expect to handle life's surprises have a clear relationship: with unwanted negativity comes pessimism or doubt that you will be able to handle the future.

In this chapter, we will be revolving around an ideology I presented in Chapter 7: getting comfortable with being uncomfortable. In fact, that's really all there is to it! The bottom line is that we have to stop treating unpredictability as a threat and start viewing it as a gift.

Growth vs Fixed Mindset

To look forward to challenges and even enjoy them, you need to have a belief instilled in yourself; the belief is that you will be able to not only handle all of life's future challenges flowing down the current, but that you will grow from them. For this belief to come to life, you will have to possess a growth mindset.

At its essence, a growth mindset is all about promoting effort, not perfection. It is not the expectation of yourself to instantaneously master every skill you set your eyes on, but rather that by applying yourself, you could make quite a bit of progress. A person with a growth mindset does not shy away from challenges because they believe that, regardless of their success, they are improving their skills. A growth mindset suggests they believe that through determination and effort, their skills and talents are capable of being improved and that they are not static.

At the other end of the spectrum, we have the concept of a fixed mindset. As the name suggests, people with a fixed mindset lack the belief that they can truly alter what they are good at. Instead, they believe that their skills and talents are more innate than anything and that challenging tasks are simply not meant for them.

Interestingly, we are all combinations of the two mindsets. If you've ever given up on something simply because it's "too hard," you've exhibited a fixed mindset. On the contrary, if you've ever put in the effort to learn something completely new to you, you've exhibited a growth mindset. A perfect growth mindset doesn't exist, as we all have both inside of us. The difference lies in the mindset we mostly rely on when faced with a challenge.

A growth mindset is more useful for absolutely any endeavor. With this perspective, you are facing the challenge head-on. Most people who exhibit this type of mindset achieve more than those who have a fixed mindset. This is not because they have better skills or anything like that, but simply because they try more new things and boldly attempt demanding tasks. After all, if you cast a wider net, you will likely get more fish!

Working On Growth

Another key component of a growth mindset that I haven't mentioned yet is accepting failure; not only that, but actively learning from your failure. If you are someone who gets intimidated by challenges quite often, you will want to learn how to transform your mindset into a growth-based one. I recommend the following useful tips on how to do so:

- Try something you've often told yourself you probably couldn't do. Maybe you've wanted to learn another language, but the magnitude of such a task scares you away from starting; or, maybe you've been wanting to start your own business. Wherever your desires may lie, it's time to let them out of their cages. It's scary, it's adrenaline-inducing, and it's inspiring, but at the end of the day, it will be worth it. So, take one small task you've been putting off because it slightly scares you, and vow to dive into it on a particular day.

- Do something badly and embrace it. This automatically goes against human nature—we don't actively strive for failure; but for the sake of your new-and-improved growth mindset, let's do exactly that. Think of an activity that you are aware you are bad at. It could be something like playing a sport, cooking a meal, writing an article, etcetera. Then, once you've done it, present it to someone for objective criticism. If you let go of your attachment to praise and validation, you open yourself up to learning from your mistakes. Starting with something simple begins training your mind to be more open to it, even on a larger scale.
- Redefine your idea of success. What is success to you? Do you have to do something near-perfectly to think of it as a success? If so, you are setting yourself up for disappointment. With a growth mindset, success is considered pure effort. By evaluating what it means to be successful to you, you might be able to change your perspective of success to include failures.

Rising to the Occasion

In many situations, success is a choice. I won't generalize and say that this is true for everyone, as there exists a lot of inequality in our society, but for many people, this should ring true. The reason so many people seemingly end up choosing wrong is because somewhere deep down, they might actually be afraid of success.

What makes a person scared of success? Well, first of all, realizing you're scared of success is not easy. Usually, it manifests as self-sabotage; an unwillingness to go after what you want, minimizing your skills and achievements. The reasons for this fear are vast, ranging from a lack of confidence to a sense of being undeserving of true success.

The first step toward overcoming something like this is breaking your history of self-sabotage, but that requires a keen sense of responsibility, and not being afraid to take accountability. Let's say you got an interview for a high-profile job that you used to wish for, but as the date for it approaches nearer and nearer, you still haven't begun preparing. Then, you wake up the day of the interview and quickly study the company and possible interview questions, just a couple of hours before. If you ended up feeling unprepared during the interview and did not get the job offer in the end, what are you blaming it on? Did you truly have no time to prepare, or was it unconscious self-sabotage pushing you to procrastinate?

If it's the latter, the truth might be a hard pill to swallow—your fear of success prevented you from believing in yourself and doing your best. However, it's better to recognize these faults and take full accountability so you prevent yourself from falling next time.

Increasing Motivation

Now, let's get to the fun part: sparking your motivation for life again. First of all, let's be clear that your zest for life comes from the motivation you have for different parts of it. In other words, you should be striving for motivation in many areas, including health, education, career, hobbies, travel, and so on.

Listening to inspiration

Inspiration often comes from other people. If there's someone you admire in a certain field, you can make a connection and ask them for some tips. If there's no one like that in your personal life, you're in luck —the internet is right at your fingertips!

I have become a massive fan of podcasts. I used to not understand the excitement of listening to people have casual conversations for half an hour or more, but then I found some that were right up my alley. I discovered podcasts about my hobbies, such as traveling, about improving mental health, career changes, and more. There are a lot of creative and successful people out there, so give them a listen! Not only does their success have the power to inspire you to want the same, but their experiences can allow you to get some additional knowledge about how to go about it.

<u>Reading content</u>

Reading is truly powerful. Although it has lost some of its popularity due to social media and other forms of content, its benefits have not decreased. If you could muster up the attention span, you could go all-in on a book. If you prefer something a little quicker to comb through, articles, blogs, and websites can present you with useful information in a very concise format.

Reading is always more enjoyable if you truly believe you're getting something out of it, whether that be entertainment or education.

<u>Setting goals</u>

When you set goals for yourself, your emotional reaction is a very telling thing. If you feel inspired when writing down your goals, you are on the right path. However, if you loathe the items on your list, perhaps it's time to make a change of path.

The method I recommend using for goal-setting is called SMART. This acronym stands for the following elements of a properly-set goal (Boogaard, 2021):

- **Specific.** A good goal diminishes vagueness as much as possible. Think about exactly what needs to be done for this goal to be achieved, and write it down. What smaller steps must be accomplished for you to get there? List everything required for this goal to become a reality.
- **Measurable.** How will you be measuring your progress? Perhaps consider a set amount of progress you want to

complete toward the goal at equal intervals of time. You should have benchmarks in place to keep track of your journey.

- **Achievable.** Let's be honest, some of us want too much, too fast. So, for this bullet point, it's time for a reality check: Can this be done? Do you have all the materials that are required for this goal? No one is saying that setting big goals is bad, but they must be realistic.
- **Relevant.** Now, evaluate how you truly feel about this goal. If you believe it will benefit your life and make you happier, then it's worth the effort. Make sure it aligns with your vision, your desires, and your values.
- **Time-bound.** A goal without an end date is simply a dream. To hold yourself accountable, set a realistic date by which you would want to achieve this goal. It can be a few weeks, months, or even years in the future.

All-in-all, motivation is a powerful tool to say goodbye to negativity bias. Without it, your negativity will get the best of you and hold you back. Things such as goal-setting, inspiration, and taking risks are all aligned with the perspective of someone who leads a positive life. Positive people embrace what life gives them with a clear mind and a heart full of passion.

Key Points

Let's look over the most important takeaways from Chapter 9:

- Our fear of being bad at something prevents us from trying and possibly succeeding
- Embracing the unpredictability of life will automatically boost your optimism
- A growth mindset is the belief that you can expand your skill set through effort
- A fixed mindset is the belief that your skill set is basically set in stone

- Becoming more open to the possibilities of the future means stepping out of your comfort zone
- Being afraid of success leads to self-sabotage, whether it's subtle or not
- Having a motivation for your life increases your satisfaction with it and consequently, your positivity

Chapter 10
Shadow Work for the Mind

"When we are aware of our weaknesses or negative tendencies, we open the opportunity to work on them."

— *Allan Lokos*

The most common solution we hear to mental health issues is therapy. Not only that, but therapy is also meant to help us through slumps, relationship issues, and problems with the way we view the world and ourselves. But, what do we do if we don't have the money for it? After all, therapy may be quite popular nowadays, but that doesn't make it any less expensive.

It's not that shadow work can replace therapy (nor should it), but it is a good alternative for someone who wants to get to the root of their issues without breaking the bank. The lack of a licensed professional present certainly makes this process a little less straightforward, but with enough honesty and vulnerability, shadow work's benefits are immeasurable.

Carl Jung—the famed Swiss psychologist—was the first to develop the concept of the shadow. He described it as the combination of repressed ideas, weaknesses, desires, instincts, and shortcomings (Cherry, 2022). The shadow is a part of all of us and is all of our ugly parts—our dark side. This part of ourselves isn't just one that we try to hide from others, but ourselves as well. Oftentimes, our shadow self can exhibit greed, envy, rage, hate, and prejudice; but, even if we don't like it, it's still there. Carl Jung believed that the shadow can show up in our dreams as various scary creatures such as snakes, demons, and dragons.

What's more interesting, however, is that the shadow self only gets bigger and stronger the longer we try to repress it. Otherwise, without coming to terms with our shadow, we allow it to make up a bigger part of ourselves. Accepting our shadow selves is no easy feat, in fact, when I first started doing shadow work, I was emotionally exhausted—but it was so worth it.

As you might've caught on, shadow work is tapping into those obscured parts of us, to establish a deeper connection to ourselves. This allows us to see ourselves for exactly who we are and why we think the way we do. Its benefits include:

- **Improved interactions with others.** The more self-aware you become, the more you trust yourself, and that kind of consciousness can be used in your relationships. For example, perhaps you were told as a child not to talk back to people, so you have trouble standing up for yourself as an adult. By doing shadow work, you can hone your boundaries and start to speak your truth.
- **Healing generational trauma.** A lot of people's families suffered terrible situations in the past that influenced generation after generation. To break this cycle, a person has to have a very strong sense of who they are and what they have to unlearn.
- **Learning healthy ways to meet your needs.** Our shadow selves can cause us to indulge in destructive behavior. For example, if a person's shadow holds within itself the idea that

wanting closeness with someone is 'clingy,' they are more likely to cheat on their partner. Through shadow work, you can identify the desires that have been manifesting in harmful behavior.

- **Gaining confidence in yourself.** Shadow work allows us to come to terms with who we are—both the good and the bad. When we become aware of our mental shortcomings, we can come to accept them and nourish them with healthy alternatives. This, in turn, gets rid of our self-doubt that an ugly side of us will come out when we least expect it. Knowing who you truly are benefits your self-esteem.
- **Improved creativity.** Your shadow doesn't just hide traits of your personality, but also skills and inclinations you may have repressed because at some point in your life you were told they shouldn't be pursued. Accepting your shadow allows you to start authentically tapping into what you truly desire.
- **Increased mental clarity.** Overall, shadow work can help you understand your thoughts, emotions, and desires. Knowing your tendencies and 'ugly' parts helps you avoid them when needed.

Ignoring your shadow self is repression. Unfortunately, not coming to terms with it can lead to issues such as:

- Substance abuse
- Mental health issues, including depression and anxiety
- Negative self-talk, including self-deprecating humor

These things occur because by ignoring your shadow self, you are not confronting what is hurting you, instead you are taking the pain out on yourself.

General Guide to Shadow Work

To properly do shadow work, the process starts before you even pick up your pen. By this, I mean that shadow work demands pure honesty.

Thankfully, you don't have to talk to anyone else about your shadow, but your honesty has to be with yourself. Good shadow work tackles the concept you have of yourself: Who are you? What do you truly want? What is holding you back?

These are three simple questions, but to get to their answers, you might have to ask yourself an abundance of other questions. I aim to write one to two pages in my journal per question, to truly dig deep for the answer. When you run out of questions, there are always more to answer. My best recommendation is to start by answering one of the following 15 questions per day (Wright, 2022):

- What do I want to get out of shadow work?
- What were my family's values? How do my values line up?
- In what ways am I like my family members? Do I hope to be similar to them or different?
- What cycles or bad habits within my family am I afraid of repeating?
- How would I describe my current life to my child self? What parts of it am I proud to tell them and which am I ashamed of?
- When was the last time I truly felt at peace? What was my environment like? Was I alone or with someone else?
- In what situations do I feel less than, equal to, or better than others?
- What is my definition of failure?
- What do I describe as my biggest personal failure? What caused it?
- When was the last time I was rejected by someone? What did I tell them?
- When was the last time I felt jealous of somebody? What about their success or personality made me feel this way? What do they have that I want?
- When was the last time I felt defensive, and what caused this?
- What behaviors in other people upset me the most? Do I exhibit any of these behaviors myself?

- How forgiving do I tend to be? Am I capable of forgiving others? What would someone have to do that is unforgivable to me?
- How do I treat myself when I do something disappointing or when I fail? Am I kind to myself or do I further beat myself down?

Meditation for the Shadow

If you ever get tired of writing and want to face your shadow directly in your mind, meditation is a wonderful alternative, and a powerful one at that. When I did my first shadow work meditation, I was nearly brought to tears, as I truly started to accept that part of myself. It took several run-throughs over the course of a few weeks for me to be totally at peace with my shadow self, but my work is still not done. You see, our shadows continue to update, re-form, and grow into new incarnations depending on our lives. So, our work with them is never really done.

I would recommend finding a guided meditation for shadow work online. For a lot of them, the guide will encourage you to visualize your shadow as yourself or even as a separate entity. By doing so, you disconnect from it and can interact with it more objectively. All of those self-doubts you harbor are easier to handle when they seem to be coming outside of your regular self.

The guided meditation will likely have you try accepting this version of yourself (or the other entity) for who they are. They might be pessimistic, mean, vengeful, and full of hate, but they still add to who we are. By learning to love this version of yourself, you are telling yourself that you are not ashamed, and don't need to hide who you are.

Talking Through the Hurt

A lot of our shadows are representations of aspects we've absorbed from other people or our interactions with them. We are often unaware of how deeply we are affected by others' words. If we have someone in our lives who brings out the worst in us, we must identify those triggers. In some cases, the people who have hurt us are no longer in our lives for one reason or another, or we simply are unable to talk to them. If this is not the case, however, talking to the person who has deeply hurt you in the past could be an extremely therapeutic process; uncomfortable, yes, but also very freeing.

The following is a guideline for beginning a conversation with someone whom you want to make peace with:

- **Understand your thoughts and feelings.** The last thing you want to do is go into such a tense situation with guns blazing. Ideally, you should have formulated a very clear picture of what exactly you feel and what you want to say.
- **Notify the person.** Each of us has good and bad days, and we need to be respectful of that. Tell the person you want to discuss something important with them and ask when would be a good time for them.
- **Find a neutral environment.** Be mindful of where and when you schedule the conversation, and make sure both of you are comfortable. Find a setting that is comfortable and not too emotional.
- **Express yourself through a three-part statement.** To not trigger the other person's defensiveness or make them feel attacked, try expressing yourself as objectively as possible. Describe what happened, how you felt about it, and what you think about it now.

Our past shapes who we are; there's no getting around it. Making peace with our past allows us to truly move forward; otherwise, you are being actively held back by what no longer even exists. This includes past people, situations, failures, rejections, and miscalculations. Yes, we can blame others, but what good would that do if it only makes us angrier? The entire premise of shadow work is to accept things for what they are, no matter how uncomfortable that may be.

Key Points

Let's look over the most important takeaways from Chapter 10:

- We all have a shadow self—the part of us that includes undesirable qualities and attributes
- Accepting and healing your shadow results in improved relationships, self-confidence, mental clarity, and more
- Journaling and answering shadow work questions daily can build your progress up bit by bit
- Meditation is a powerful technique to visualize and accept your shadow self
- You can't fix the past, but you should address it, especially if somebody has hurt you

Conclusion

There is not a single person who can escape the difficulties caused by negativity. We all struggle, face obstacles, fail, get upset, and sometimes even give up. Success doesn't come easy, but the effort put toward it is worthwhile if what you're working for is truly what you desire. Negativity is no joke and rarely does it ease up on its own. However, through introspection, mindfulness, shadow work, and motivation increase, you can prevent yourself from being swiped down by the avalanche of negativity.

If there is one thing I want you to take away from this book, it's that your negative thoughts should not be your enemies. They exist for a very specific and helpful reason—to help you navigate this crazy world—and it's only when you let them go from insightful guides to overpowering rulers that they become a venom in your life. If those little voices in your head become so deafening that they overshadow all the positive things in your life—including all the things that pose no real threat to you—then it's imperative that you learn to adjust their volume; because, if you try to just tune them out, chances are they will not go away anytime soon.

When your negative thoughts make up the majority of what goes on inside your brain, it's a losing battle to start countering them with positive thoughts, since they will be few and far between at first. The best thing to do is to take the power away from the pre-existing negative thoughts, rather than just conjuring up new, positive ones. For that, you can:

- Look objectively at your negative thoughts and feelings, and accept them without judgment
- Try to get to the bottom of why they appear, what they mean to you, as well as what they mean to your situation
- Let them go gradually, by learning to live with them, but without letting them cause you much pain until eventually they stop coming
- Be kinder to yourself and work on your self-image. None of us are perfect, so don't strive to be
- Improve other areas of your life that will make you a happier person by using various techniques

Remember, you are in control of your inner dialogue, so you must be mindful of what's going on inside your head. By being aware of the path your subconscious might be leading you down, you can change which way you go. You have the power to decide what is true to you, and what you consider to be the most helpful interpretation, at all times.

Positivity is much more unnatural to us than negativity is, so naturally, it will take some extra work for us to become comfortable with it. I promise you, however, that the benefits you reap will prove to be worth it. By making your mind a safe place rather than one of critique and doubting, you begin growing into someone you are not only comfortable being, but are proud of. So, take accountability for your future and don't put off your happiness any longer.

I hope with all my heart that this book was of use to you. Keep in mind that not all of the techniques I shared will resonate with you; it's for this reason that I provided a multitude of various exercises, techniques, and questions to ask yourself so that you can create a method that works just for you. With over a decade of experience, I learned precisely how important it is to try various things out until something sticks.

Thankfully, you won't ever be short of options. Not only do you now have ten chapters of information from me, but countless articles, studies, and educational materials, are being constantly updated online nowadays. With pure intentions and a fiery determination to improve your life, I am confident you will be just fine.

Bibliography

150+ mindfulness quotes to help you live more mindfully. Declutter The Mind. (2021, September 14). Retrieved July 15, 2022, from https://declutterthemind.com/blog/mindfulness-quotes/

175 feel-good happiness quotes: Keep inspiring me. KeepInspiring.me. (2022, June 28). Retrieved July 15, 2022, from https://www.keepinspiring.me/quotes-about-happiness/

44% of students don't know what they want to do after graduation. Concrete. (2015, February 8). Retrieved July 15, 2022, from https://www.concrete-online.co.uk/44-students-dont-know-want-graduation/

Allen, S., & Smith, J. A. (2016). *How happy brains respond to negative things*. Greater Good. Retrieved July 15, 2022, from https://greatergood.berkeley.edu/article/item/how_happy_brains_respond_to_negative_things

Bergeron, L. (2013, November 20). *Size, connectivity of brain region linked to anxiety level in young children, study shows*. News Center. Retrieved July 15, 2022, from https://med.stanford.edu/news/all-news/2013/11/size-connectivity-of-brain-region-linked-to-anxiety-level-in-young-children-study-shows.html

Bloom, L. B. (2022, April 14). *Ranked: The 20 happiest countries in the world in 2022*. Forbes. Retrieved July 15, 2022, from https://www.forbes.com/sites/laurabegleybloom/2022/03/18/ranked-the-20-happiest-countries-in-the-world-in-2022/?sh=5e975d9835d5

Boogaard, K. (2022, February 17). *How to write SMART goals*. Work Life by Atlassian. Retrieved July 15, 2022, from https://www.atlassian.com/blog/productivity/how-to-write-smart-goals

Cherry, K. (2022, May 2). *Which Jungian archetype are you?* Verywell Mind. Retrieved July 15, 2022, from https://www.verywellmind.com/what-are-jungs-4-major-archetypes-2795439#:~:text=The%20shadow%20is%20an%20archetype,to%20cultural%20norms%20and%20expectations.

Clear, J. (2020, February 4). *Inversion: The crucial thinking skill nobody ever taught you*. James Clear. Retrieved July 15, 2022, from https://jamesclear.com/inversion

Congleton, C., Holzel, B. K., & Lazar, S. W. (2021, August 30). *Mindfulness can literally change your brain*. Harvard Business Review. Retrieved July 15, 2022, from https://hbr.org/2015/01/mindfulness-can-literally-change-your-brain#:~:text=Neuroscientists%20have%20also%20shown%20that,thinking%2C%20and%20sense%20of%20self.

Danzico, M. (2011, April 24). *Brains of Buddhist monks scanned in meditation study*. BBC News. Retrieved July 15, 2022, from https://www.bbc.com/news/world-us-canada-12661646

Divorce statistics and facts: What affects divorce rates in the U.S.? Wilkinson & Finkbeiner, LLP. (2022, March 3). Retrieved July 30, 2022, from https://www.wf-lawyers.com/divorce-statistics-and-facts/#:~:text=Almost%2050%20percent%20of%20all,8.

Geggel, L. (2020, March 17). *Meditation may have shaved 8 years of aging off Buddhist monk's brain*. LiveScience. Retrieved July 15, 2022, from https://www.livescience.com/buddhist-monk-meditation-brain.html

Gjersoe, N. (2017, May 26). *Negativity bias: Why Conservatives are more swayed by threats than Liberals*. The Guardian. Retrieved July 15, 2022, from https://www.theguardian.com/science/head-quarters/2017/may/26/negativity-bias-why-conservatives-are-more-swayed-by-threats-than-liberals

Goodreads. (n.d.). *A quote by C.S. Lewis*. Goodreads. Retrieved July 15, 2022, from https://www.goodreads.com/quotes/812245-you-are-never-too-old-to-set-another-goal-or

Goodreads. (n.d.). *A quote by Wayne W. Dyer*. Goodreads. Retrieved July 15, 2022, from https://www.goodreads.com/quotes/126097-what-we-think-determines-what-happens-to-us-so-if

Goodreads. (n.d.). *Overthinking quotes (151 quotes)*. Goodreads. Retrieved July 15, 2022, from https://www.goodreads.com/quotes/tag/overthinking

Goodreads. (n.d.). *Shirley MacLaine quotes (author of out on a limb)*. Goodreads. Retrieved July 15, 2022, from https://www.goodreads.com/author/quotes/63879.Shirley_MacLaine#:~:text=%E2%80%9CDwelling%20on%20the%20negative%20simply%20contributes%20to%20its%20power.%E2%80%9D

Goss, R. (2022, January 26). *This island unlocked the secret to long life-and knows how to get through tough times*. Travel. Retrieved July 15, 2022, from https://www.nationalgeographic.com/travel/article/uncover-the-secrets-of-longevity-in-this-japanese-village

Inspirational quotes about history...and the future. Everyday Power. (2022, July 10). Retrieved July 15, 2022, from https://everydaypower.com/history-quotes/

Inspiring quotes on getting rid of bad habits. Everyday Power. (2022, June 3). Retrieved July 15, 2022, from https://everydaypower.com/quotes-getting-rid-of-bad-habits/

Klemp, N. (2019, August 7). *The neuroscience of breaking out of negative thinking (and how to do it in under 30 seconds)*. Inc.com. Retrieved July 15, 2022, from https://www.inc.com/nate-klemp/try-this-neuroscience-based-technique-to-shift-your-mindset-from-negative-to-positive-in-30-seconds.html

Kondo, M. (2014). *The Life-Changing Magic of Tidying up*. Ten Speed Press.

Kondo, M. (2021, August 14). *The joy of sleep, with Arianna Huffington – konmari: The official website of Marie Kondo*. KonMari. Retrieved July 15, 2022, from https://konmari.com/arianna-huffington-sleep/

Lewis, M. (2016, November 14). *How two trailblazing psychologists turned the world of decision science upside down*. Vanity Fair. Retrieved July 15, 2022, from https://www.vanityfair.com/news/2016/11/decision-science-daniel-kahneman-amos-tversky

Mcleod, S. (2020, December 29). *Maslow's hierarchy of needs*. Simply Psychology. Retrieved July 15, 2022, from https://www.simplypsychology.org/maslow.html

Shadow self quotes: Thought-provoking sayings about inner darkness. SOLANCHA. (2020, August 14). Retrieved July 15, 2022, from https://solancha.com/shadow-self-quotes-thought-provoking-sayings-about-inner-darkness/

Tracy, B. (n.d.). *Excerpt from get smart!* Penguin Random House Canada. Retrieved July 15, 2022, from https://www.penguinrandomhouse.ca/books/533286/get-smart-by-brian-tracy/9780399183799/excerpt

Why does your brain love? negativity? the negativity bias. Marbella International University Centre. (2021, June 10). Retrieved July 15, 2022, from https://miuc.org/brain-love-

negativity-negativity-bias/#:~:text=Much%20research%20has%20been%20-
done,known%20to%20cause%20neutral%20feelings.

Wilson, T. D., & Gilbert, D. T. (2005, June 1). *Affective forecasting: Knowing what to want - sage journals*. Sage Journals. Retrieved July 15, 2022, from https://journals.sagepub.-com/doi/10.1111/j.0963-7214.2005.00355.x

Wright, J. (2022, January 12). *30 shadow work prompts for healing and growth*. PureWow. Retrieved July 15, 2022, from https://www.purewow.com/wellness/shadow-work-prompts

Xplore. (n.d.). *Aristotle quotes*. BrainyQuote. Retrieved July 15, 2022, from https://www.brainyquote.com/quotes/aristotle_138768

Xplore. (n.d.). *Benjamin Franklin quotes*. BrainyQuote. Retrieved July 15, 2022, from https://www.brainyquote.com/authors/benjamin-franklin-quotes

Set Good Boundaries

Where You Stop, and I Begin

Introduction

We all have a deep need for belonging and feeling connected to others. Human nature predisposes us to form bonds of attachment. It's a survival instinct and one of the most powerful dynamics between humans that has allowed us to multiply and thrive. Parents have a primal understanding that they must care for their child if it is to survive. A child naturally forms an attachment to the caregiver who ensures its survival needs are met. This is the first deep human connection we establish and, as we grow, this primal need for attachment evolves. As Brené Brown describes beautifully in the quote above, we are hardwired for attachment and a sense of belonging.

But attachment is not the only fundamental need we have as humans. As children, and later as adults, we have an equally important desire for authenticity. Authenticity is about recognizing your own strengths, accepting who you are, and having the courage and self-confidence to share this with the world. This is where boundaries come in. Boundaries define us. They protect our time, energy, health, and peace. They aren't about keeping things out, but about protecting what's inside.

When these two fundamental needs (attachment and authenticity) are completely in balance, we can be genuinely supportive of others without sacrificing our own needs. In many cases, however, we choose attachment (or approval and recognition from others) over authenticity. We, understandably, deem it more important for others to like us than to speak our truth. Frankly, it can be easier to sweep our thoughts, feelings, and desires under the rug in an effort to please the people around us.

We are in a constant dilemma to be authentic while at the same time trying to nurture our attachment to others. This interplay between authenticity and our primal need for attachment is where tension arises and our vision gets blurred when it comes to setting healthy boundaries.

Boundaries aren't like physical borders around countries—we can't see them, touch them, or run into them, so how do we make sure they're there? Knowing ourselves and communicating with others is a great start. We have to be aware of our metaphorical on-and-off switch: What makes us feel good in a relationship and what makes us feel bad? The problem often lies in the fact that people feel more comfortable bending their own boundaries to satisfy someone else's needs, rather than simply telling them 'no'. It is only through understanding the importance of boundaries that we will be able to actually take that step. Otherwise, we will continue living in our comfort zones, allowing others to take advantage of our kindness, time, and energy. If we don't set boundaries for ourselves, someone else will set them for us. We will agree to things we don't want to do, give up our autonomy, and forfeit our own satisfaction. And in the worst case, we lose touch with our true selves.

It's easy to blame others for taking more than they give, but we must learn to take control of our own destiny. Setting boundaries is key to safeguarding your authentic self, but if we are to master the craft of saying "no" more often, we must first examine the reasons why we limit ourselves in this way.

Establishing boundaries in your relationships isn't a change that can be made overnight. It takes time to build up your confidence, courage, and willpower to establish and clearly express your limits. Our unique experiences, preferences, and morals influence the way we want our relationships to be. These aspects require some deep self-reflection in order for us to become aware of our boundaries and adjust our relationships accordingly.

By declaring that our happiness is in our own hands, we transfer that responsibility onto ourselves. It might seem scary to realize the success of your life depends on you, but it is the better alternative. It allows you to take the steps—no matter how difficult—to stop letting others drain you.

Boundaries will open up a whole new chapter of your life that you might have been deprived of this whole time. They will make space for you to live the life you want and cultivate relationships that allow you to grow into the best version of yourself.

By the end of this book, you will have all the tools you need to start enjoying the countless benefits of having carved out space for YOU to thrive. To list a few:

- Increased independence and gaining happiness and fulfillment from within
- Improved self-esteem
- Ability to focus on your own well-being
- Allow your authentic needs space to thrive
- Prevent being taken advantage of by others
- Become more assertive and say 'no' when needed
- Prevent social/relationship burnout

The list goes on and on. Boundaries are essential. Your life is likely shaped by boundaries you may not even be aware of. This book is about much more than simply teaching you to say 'no' - it is meant to help you understand the complex dynamics at play in all your relationships and free you from the burden of pleasing others.

Chapter 1
What are Boundaries?

"Each time you set a healthy boundary, you say 'yes' to more freedom."

— *Nancy Levin*

Some people define boundaries as our basic moral compass. This means they would include rules such as no cheating, no lying, respecting others' time by not being late to events, or being honest about your feelings. To others, boundaries cover aspects that are less about moral standards and more about personal preferences. The foundation of any healthy relationship consists of comfort, safety, and trust. These three aspects look different depending on whom you ask, so to understand how to establish boundaries, you must first evaluate what things have to be in place in order for you to feel secure and happy in your relationships.

Many people will base their boundaries around some of their previous experiences. If they were often yelled at as a child, then being yelled at by other people (even as an adult) can trigger some harmful memories and bring up feelings of being unsafe. Yelling is usually a red flag in any relationship—it demonstrates a lack of respect, an inability to control emotions, and a failure to participate in mature conversations. However, to some people, yelling is considerably more traumatizing and much more of a deal breaker than it is to others. Some people wouldn't cut a friend off just because they raised their voice a few times, but other people certainly would.

Another example could be a friendship or relationship where one wants to spend a lot of time together while the other person feels smothered. Some people simply *love* to surround themselves with people all the time while others place a greater value on their alone time or doing things independently.

This goes to show that boundaries aren't solely representative of the morals you hold. It doesn't have to be only about what you believe is right and wrong—it can also be simply about how you want to be treated.

Types of Boundaries

Let's get into the thick of it and explore the different forms of boundaries. There are seven different types (Martin, 2020):

1. **Physical boundaries.** Physical boundaries are meant to provide you with a safe space. They range anywhere from being entitled to basic resources such as food and water, to specific things that make you feel secure. Asking people to not open your closet is a physical boundary, as is asking people to not sit too close to you. Physical boundaries convey that you are the *only one* who gets to decide how your body and personal space can be treated.
2. **Sexual boundaries.** These boundaries can be of sexual or romantic nature. Due to its naturally touchy subject, many people are very well aware of what sexual boundaries they have but are scared to communicate and maintain them. Sexual boundaries should cover everything you *are* and *aren't*

comfortable with; in other words, how far you are willing to go sexually. For example: how often you are willing to have sex, what positions you are and aren't willing to try out, and how and where you would like to be touched or not. Sexual boundaries should be very firm and completely understood by your partner(s); make sure to prevent any possible grey areas and get very clear on your preferences and limits with each other. Don't forget that sexual boundaries can be dynamic. You might suddenly feel uncomfortable and change your mind, and that's perfectly fine.

3. **Emotional and mental boundaries.** With emotional and mental boundaries (lumped together into one single category), you are effectively taking power over your thoughts and feelings; seems like this is a given fact, right? Well, these boundaries go beyond just stating the obvious. They form the barrier between your own emotions and the emotions experienced by others. In other words, while you are responsible for how you are feeling, you are not responsible for how others feel. This applies to many situations, including those in which the behavior of someone else makes you feel unpleasant. For example, if your sibling likes to one-up you every time you express your feelings, you could kindly explain to them that their experience does not invalidate yours. Another instance could be if someone always dumps their trauma on you as a form of 'friendship bonding'—you could let them know that while you understand their experience, you cannot be emotionally responsible to console them at all times. Their pain is not your burden to bear.

4. **Spiritual and religious boundaries.** Spiritual and religious boundaries go both ways: for the person that has faith in a set of beliefs as well as for the person that does not hold that same faith. If you are a religious or spiritual person, the people you hold relationships with should respect that and allow you to believe and practice your faith even if they do not. On the flip side, if you are not a religious or spiritual person and someone in your life cannot accept that, they will likely try over and over

again to push their personal beliefs onto you. In this case, you are also entitled to set a religious boundary by making it clear that you want them to stop trying to change your belief system.

5. **Financial and material boundaries.** Money is the root of all evil, right? Well, I would disagree. I say that what money does to people is the root of all evil and not the money itself. In a lot of cases, money is indeed the root of many problems in family relationships, romantic relationships, and even friendships. Financial boundaries allow you to be in full control of your finances: where you want to spend your money, how you want to earn it, whom you want to lend it to, and how much you want to save. With this boundary, you are not allowing others to treat your money as their own. The same concept is applied to material boundaries—you are the only one who ultimately decides how a material object of yours gets to be treated. Examples could look like saying "No, I cannot lend you another $1,000," or "Please, ask me first before you borrow my laptop."

6. **Time boundaries.** In my belief, time is the most valuable resource of all since we can't get it back, no matter how hard we try. For this reason, we should be putting extra care into making sure that our time stays ours. To nourish and maintain equal relationships you must keep full ownership of your time. Setting a time boundary will prevent those around you from exploiting it. You could tell your friend that you cannot hang out with them all weekend because you have other things to do. The same can be applied if someone always asks you to help them with tasks over and over again—your time is yours and it is okay to say no, even if you don't have a clear reason.

7. **Non-negotiable boundaries.** Non-negotiable boundaries are a category of their own, but they are often one of the previously mentioned six types. The name might speak for itself, but non-negotiable boundaries are those that signify a dealbreaker for a relationship. Non-negotiable boundaries make us feel safe. If you are a monogamous person and your

partner cheats on you, they have likely broken a non-negotiable boundary. If your friend refuses to be careful while driving, you will probably stop getting into a car with them. The people in your life should be aware of the concrete non-negotiable boundaries you have. We must be careful not to place too many of our boundaries in this category. You must be prepared to stick to your non-negotiables for them to have any significance.

As you start to get a sense of these various types of boundaries, you can begin to examine your own. In a lot of cases, people prevent themselves from exploring what is possible when it comes to boundaries. Many of us have been taught from a young age that certain boundaries are invalid or selfish. We will explore this further in the next few chapters, but there is nothing narcissistic and self-serving about setting boundaries with those around you.

Knowing What to Look For

Many people who did not grow up being meticulously taught about boundaries (so, most of us) are likely to interpret them as something cold when in reality, "maintaining boundaries is about being the gate-keeper of your life in order to keep yourself safe and well," (Nitka, 2020). What many people don't realize is that they already have boundaries that are unique to them. They are simply unaware of what exactly those boundaries are, and as such find themselves unable to communicate them effectively to others.

Mina was a client of mine. She had a longtime friend, Richard, with a short fuse. From the sounds of it, you wouldn't want to be near Richard when his anger took over, and he had become prone to directing his rage toward Mina during heartfelt conversations. Mina ruminated as to how her friend could suddenly become so cruel toward her. This crossed a line, but she wasn't sure how to address it after so many years of friendship. They had always mended the relationship after such episodes and she had never felt threatened by him, but Mina had reached the end of her rope and was considering cutting all ties. Experience tells me there is likely some trauma lurking underneath explosive outbursts of rage, so we dug deeper.

Understanding the root of her friend's behavior was the first step toward Mina feeling empowered to assert herself. Exploring what provoked Richard, it became clear that his anger typically surfaced while he was airing out conflicts in his life and Mina asked questions to better understand his situation. Mina was showing she cared enough to learn more, yet he felt interrogated. Mina wanted to understand her friend but all he needed was to feel unconditionally supported. While there is a lot more to unpack here, this example points to the importance of understanding one's own boundaries.

There seemed to be a mental-emotional boundary Richard was unaware of, which led him to lash out. When he lashed out, he violated a strict boundary of Mina's, but she was hesitant to address this because she felt at fault. It wasn't necessary to determine *why* Mina's questions triggered his rage; it was enough to acknowledge that Mina could not carry on in this relationship as long as she continued to be treated this way.

Mina, armed with the awareness that this wasn't about *her* but rather about Richard's inability to control his behavior, Mina confronted the issue with her longtime friend. By communicating her own boundary, she found out that Richard had been perceiving Mina's questions as intruding on his space. He lashed out irrationally in an unnecessary defense. She placed a limit on what she would tolerate, and in doing so uncovered the trigger point of a boundary Richard had been unaware of. This didn't solve the problem overnight, but Mina had opened up the floor for an important conversation that had the power to change their relationship going forward.

Boundaries exist whether you acknowledge them or not. Maybe you don't like being hugged, maybe you feel ignored if your friend doesn't reply to a text message for several days, or perhaps you don't like discussing a certain triggering topic in conversation. We don't necessarily have to create or think up our boundaries, but rather we need to look deep within ourselves to uncover or rediscover them.

The People Who Are Good for You

We can't negate the impact people can have on our personal growth, no matter how good or bad their intentions may be. The list below serves as a good litmus test for healthy interpersonal relationships. Do a quick inventory of the people closest to you. Are your relationships with them characterized by the qualities below?

- **They are genuinely happy for you.** This one ought to be non-negotiable. If the people around you are not genuinely happy for you most of the time, they are not in this relationship for the right reasons. Do they help you celebrate your successes or does their reaction come from a place of insecurity or jealousy? Do they attribute your accomplishments to dumb luck or are they encouraging and supportive? You should not be hearing comments that negate your achievements or belittle your dreams. Constant attempts to keep you small are warning signs that someone does not have your best interest at heart.
- **They are there for you when times are rough.** It's easy to spend time with someone when both of your lives are running smoothly. What happens when things get tough? Can you rely on the support of those around you? Do you feel part of a community that has your back? When people who care about us know that we are going through a difficult time, they make themselves emotionally available for the sake of our well-being. This could come in the form of calling to check in, offering to help with an errand, or simply being there when you need to vent.
- **They are dependable and stick to their word.** Things come up, emergencies happen, and moods can change—that's understandable. You should, however, feel able to rely on the people in your life. Do they usually show up on time? Are they responsive when you reach out? What we're looking for is predictable and generally consistent behavior. Trust is a powerful bonding agent and having people around who we

trust to be dependable makes us feel safe, stable, and part of a strong community.

- **They respect your differences.** Respecting another person's differences displays acceptance of their authenticity. We might not always see eye to eye with the people closest to us, but we must appreciate or try to understand their points of view. It should feel safe to disagree, and you should feel comfortable discussing your interests. Curiosity in another person's interests is a primary building block that fuels connection and deepens the bond over time.
- **They don't hold you back.** People should celebrate your success, inspire you to move forward with things that interest you, and generally support your growth. Those around you should inspire you to have faith in yourself and continuously improve your life. Someone who is stuck in a rut of their own will drain the energy and suck the motivation out of everyone around them, even without intending to do so. They may elicit your urge to enable their bad behaviors. Nobody is responsible for what life throws at them, but we all must take ownership of our path forward. Misery loves company, so don't get sucked into the vortex of another's downward spiral.

Any violation of the above is a red flag signaling the need for clearly defined boundaries in that relationship. Just as a seed needs sun and water to sprout, we must find ourselves in a supportive environment as we embark on this journey of personal growth.

Let me tell you this: surrounding yourself with the right people can change everything. Once we realize the weight of other people's influence on our lives, we can use that in our favor by pursuing new relationships that propel us toward better versions of ourselves. I have seen my life change drastically by surrounding myself with people I look up to. I began opening myself up to those who were more experienced than me or had already achieved what I wanted to achieve. Not only did their influence convince me that my dreams were realistic, but their example gave me a blueprint on how to achieve my goals.

Key Takeaways

- Boundaries are meant to create a relationship that both parties feel safe and happy in.
- Necessary boundaries will vary from person to person.
- There are seven general types of boundaries that cover different aspects of relationships.
- Our boundaries influence our relationships, whether we are aware of them or not.
- The first step in deciding which relationships in your life are worth nourishing is identifying how those people make you feel.
- People who are worth your time and energy will be happy for your success, support you when times are tough, and are dedicated to respecting you.

Chapter 2
Assessing Your Current Boundaries

The only real conflict you will ever have in your life won't be with others, but with yourself.

— Shannon L. Alder

Before we get to the meat of setting good boundaries, let's examine the boundaries already at work in your current relationships. Healthy boundaries give you space to be yourself. They protect what's inside yet allow others in only to the extent you permit. Not all boundaries are healthy, however. It is possible that some of the boundaries you already have in place could be doing more harm than good. If you feel a sense of anger or resentment, or you're simply overwhelmed in any of your relationships, there's a good chance that unhealthy boundaries are at play.

The Irony of Trust

As said by author Patrick Lencioni (2010), "teamwork begins by building trust. And the only way to do that is to overcome our need for invulnerability." A beautiful quote that captures the essence of forming boundaries: letting go of fear while ensuring your trust won't be abused.

Trust issues are a massively complex setback in relationships and can severely interfere with setting healthy boundaries. I'd argue that many of us have trust issues to one extent or another. This comes down to the fact that trust is not the safe option, and people need to feel safe.

In all transparency, trust isn't always safe. Relationships of any kind are guided by our intuition when we choose to trust, but there is likely one point or another in all our lives where our trust was misplaced. Think of people who get married to the love of their life only to be cheated on 11 years down the line or someone's childhood friend dramatically cutting ties out of the blue. Even good people make bad choices. We simply cannot predict or control other people's behavior.

On the one hand, having too much trust in others can cause you to get hurt by having boundaries that are too loose. On the other hand, having barely any trust in others means your boundaries are likely to be so rigid you never let others get close enough to truly know you. Examining your own propensity to trust and how that is interlinked with your boundaries is key to helping you better assess some areas for improvement.

An interesting 2006 study by psychologists Janine Willis and Alexander Todorov showed that people make the initial decision to trust someone within a mere 100 milliseconds of examining their face. Shocking, right? This means our brains have made up a brief template of what a trustworthy face might look like and manage to match it in real life within only a fraction of a second. We have a built-in system that can make a quick assessment of whether to trust a person or not. Based on life experience we adapt this mechanism and our risk assessment becomes more fine-tuned. Sadly, if our trust has been betrayed to extreme degrees or too many times, we are likely to look suspiciously at any new person in our lives and tend to keep others at a safe distance.

A major reason people are hesitant to set boundaries is that they view them as barriers or tools used to keep people at arm's length. Contrary to that notion, when you form a clear boundary you are in fact inviting them in, on your terms. By sharing your values with that person, you are giving them a tool to nurture a relationship with you. This creates a safe space for you to be open and vulnerable with each other, which is essential for any relationship to flourish. Boundaries are not about shutting people out at all; they are an essential part of strong relationships.

The irony of trust lies in its necessity. To form those deep, enriching connections with others we have to have trust. Yet, it's the one thing that can hurt us the most if it comes to be betrayed. So, how do we motivate ourselves to trust someone after getting burned?

Do It for You!

There's one crucial thing we all must accept: living with a constant guard up, neck-deep in trust issues, is a much more boring life to endure than one that's filled with a genuine openness and some occasional heartbreaks.

Forgiveness and trust have some key commonalities. We tend to think of these actions as something we give to others who we deem worthy or deserving of them. Interestingly enough, trust and forgiveness have more to do with ourselves and our inner peace. Neither is emotionally easy and both make us feel vulnerable to our core. It's not easy to trust again after a betrayal, nor is it always palatable to forgive someone who has caused deep pain.

"To forgive is to set a prisoner free and discover that the prisoner was you," said Lewis B. Smedes, and he could not have put it better. Of course, choosing to trust again and forgiving one's past betrayals are not synonymous, but they are certainly correlated. Through forgiveness, you tell yourself it's okay to finally let go of that hurt. It could be as simple as you needing to forgive yourself for trusting someone that ultimately hurt you. If you aren't ready to forgive another person for something they did, at least be willing to liberate yourself from the burden of pain it caused. It is about finding acceptance for what happened, leaving history in the past, and allowing yourself to move on.

The Power of Being Vulnerable

Entertainment media and even our everyday interactions prove that society at large still portrays vulnerability as a weakness. Many of us are taught to keep our vulnerabilities hidden away so as not to be taken advantage of. Because of the possibility of rejection or failure, we tend to perceive vulnerability as a risky endeavor. Any time we make ourselves vulnerable, we are taking the risk of an intense emotional response due to the higher stakes involved. However, if no one ever introduced a wild idea that was sure to be shot down, we wouldn't have achieved any of the innovations that make modern life so comfortable.

I used to consult with an individual named Ashley. She prided herself on being outspoken and had earned the respect of her colleagues, but had become stuck in a cycle of limiting herself after some recent ideas had been brushed off. Ashley displayed vulnerability by proposing creative ideas and felt defeated when they were disregarded by her team. Her knee-jerk reaction was to muzzle herself and support an idea proposed by a teammate instead.

I wanted to delve deeper into Ashley's mindset so I asked her what might have been lackluster about her proposals. Were they impractical? Did they fail to address the team's goal? What roadblocks had she over-looked that would derail her plan? Why might her colleagues have disre-garded the ideas in question? Through our conversations, it became clear that Ashley had a big-picture idea but had been watering it down to conform with the expected reaction from her team. She didn't want to ruffle any feathers or dream too big. Essentially, Ashley - the poster child of displaying vulnerability - was still limiting herself. We concluded that her proposals were solid and, rather than muzzling herself, Ashley needed to become *more* vulnerable and communicate her full proposal. She was treating her vulnerability as a weakness, but it was clear to me that her fearlessness to speak up was a trait her colleagues admired about her and it had allowed her to grow to this point in her career.

Ashley strutted into our next meeting looking victorious. She had made peace with her recent defeat and reintroduced her proposal, this time confidently presenting the full picture and elaborating on the details that would give the proposal wings to fly. She was praised for her outside-the-box approach and the team agreed to move forward with the first phase of her plan.

Being vulnerable isn't a sign of weakness, it is a sign of courage and lies at the basis of authentic connections. Ironically, it's only when we're able to establish healthy boundaries that we can fully appreciate the positive sides of vulnerability.

The Side-effects of Unhealthy Boundaries

We've discussed some of the positive effects of setting boundaries, but what happens when we *don't* set them? What are the side effects?

Generally, having poor boundaries will lead to resentment, anger, and burnout. The consequences of not setting healthy boundaries often include stress, feeling overwhelmed, financial problems, wasted time, and relationship issues, all of which have a great impact on our well-being.

Many people who are suffering from a lack of boundaries in their relationships don't even recognize why they feel so bad. I know too many people who have become victims of this. Their time was exploited, their personal belongings and safety were violated, and oftentimes their emotional state was not even considered. They knew they felt awful, but they didn't know *why*.

When your boundaries are either too loose or too rigid, your needs go unmet. This can lead to dissatisfaction and ultimately to anxiety, losing touch with yourself, and even depression. People with boundaries that are too loose often report difficulty identifying their own emotions and needs. Let's say you are overly agreeable and frequently suppress your own opinions in deference to the opinions of others. There reaches a point where you may lose sight of the line that separates your authentic self from the mask you put on to relate with the people in your life. Becoming over-involved in other people's lives, perfectionism, people-pleasing, and taking on excessive amounts of commitments are all common symptoms pointing to a lack of healthy boundaries.

Boundaries that are too rigid often come from a fear of losing your freedom and independence, which leads to feelings of emptiness and loneliness. Boundaries that are too rigid stem from the paradoxical interplay between a desire for connection and the dread of intimacy. Rigid boundaries safeguard your vulnerability, keeping it locked away.

In our journey toward setting healthy boundaries, it is important to make sure our current (and future) boundaries are not too loose and not too rigid.

Recognizing Unhealthy Boundaries

Let's look at some situations people with poor boundaries find themselves in:

- *Feeling disrespected in your relationships.* A person who makes you feel disrespected is not necessarily doing so out of hatred—more often than not, they do not recognize how their actions are making you feel. If your husband thinks you don't have an issue with him leaving dirty dishes on the counter, he will continue to do so.
- *Feeling unsafe in your relationships.* A person's behavior should never trigger a sense of danger within you. Likewise, you should not feel the relationship is at stake if you refuse to go along with someone's demands. Feeling safe speaks not just to physical danger, but your emotional stability and well-being should not be threatened either.
- *Emotions of jealousy and envy.* If you are with someone who is naturally flirty, you might understand what I'm talking about. Let's say your partner is a flirt but you are well aware that they have no intention of betraying your relationship. They love you, but their flirtatiousness gets the best of them. Even if you know your partner is like this, you might find this style of communication troubling. By not speaking up, you give your

partner space to continue flirting with others, and you will continue to suffer in silence. Which sounds harder: enduring mind-numbing jealousy every time the two of you go out or having one potentially awkward, yet honest conversation?

- *Struggle to be there for others in a meaningful way.* When you are expected to give an inordinate amount of your time to a few people in your life, how will you be able to be there for others? Your automatic, unconscious response to someone wanting to spend time with you might be a sense of dread. You likely feel spread too thin and struggle to be emotionally present in many of your relationships. It is difficult to form connections founded on mutual respect.

- *Lower self-esteem.* Not only does your self-esteem suffer when you are being treated with less respect than you deserve, but this can be augmented by the fact that you are suppressing your authenticity. If you stop being able to be happy in certain relationships, you often have to fake it. For example, you may find yourself constantly going along with the unusual demands of a friend or relative, eventually convincing yourself it makes you happy to appease them. This lack of genuineness often makes people start to dislike themselves, seeing as they are, in essence, not living out their truth.

- *Feeling numb.* Numbness is a consequence of poor boundaries that tends to occur after a long period of time. The longer you go without setting boundaries, the less likely you are to set them. We start losing touch with what we want and need, feel empty, and don't know who we are anymore. It's a feeling of being so deep in the trenches you may as well not bother climbing out.

Key Takeaways

- You cannot have healthy relationships unless you have a healthy trust level—too little or too much of it can cause your boundaries to be either too rigid or too loose.

- Do not let your painful experiences in the past hold control over your present and future relationships.
- Willingness to express vulnerability is essential to forming strong bonds.
- Resentment, anger, and feeling overwhelmed are some key indicators that firmer boundaries need to be applied.

Chapter 3
What's Needed for Boundaries?

"Boundaries protect the things that are of value to you. They keep you in alignment with what you have decided you want in life. That means the key to good boundaries is knowing what you want."

— Adelyn Birch

Setting boundaries is difficult! I get it. In fact, I've *lived* it. But if we don't establish boundaries, other people won't know how to interact with us. We'll end up feeling disrespected and misunderstood. On top of that, we may start to resent others when we're unable to recognize our own boundaries.

Let's take a quick look at an example: You are living with your romantic partner who you've been with for several years now. The honeymoon phase is over, you are both very comfortable in each other's presence and you consider your relationship to be a loving one overall. You both work full-time jobs with somewhat different schedules, contributing pretty equally to your household's finances. Now, imagine that you are beginning to notice your counterpart is doing far less around the house than you. Let's say they end work at four in the afternoon, but you're done at nine. You regularly come home after a long day at work and find your partner sitting amongst a pile of unfolded laundry, or a stack of dirty dishes from breakfast remains in the sink. You're exhausted from your day and would rather not initiate a conversation about this, so you do these chores yourself.

This scenario tends to set off little red flags for most people because we are primed to expect a degree of reciprocity in our relationships. This feeling of disappointment and being let down by your partner may challenge your sense of self-worth. When someone is not pulling their weight with the simple things, you may question their ability to meaningfully contribute to the relationship when it matters most.

Now, do you think this person is leaving chores for you out of malice or ill intent? I doubt the answer is yes, however it is more important to first examine your reaction to the emotions that come about when someone lets you down. Beyond assigning an assumed reason for the bad behavior, how does it make you feel? Are there larger aspects of the relationship that this small household chore might call into question? Get clear on what it is about the neglected chores that sets you off. It is exactly these things that need to be addressed when you confront your partner with the issue.

You see, if this is a healthy relationship, you will probably have to go through a conversation or two to set this boundary straight. Boundaries are not a form of harsh ultimatums nor are they meant to sour the vibe between two people. They are simply a definition of your limits, encouraging others to keep them in mind.

Instead of starting a conversation about your partner not pulling their weight, a more effective approach would sound more like "Honey, when you do x, it makes me feel y". Expressing those feelings calls on you to be vulnerable, which signals that you care enough to solve the issue rather than revert to anger or the blame game. By getting better at addressing the root cause of the problem at hand you will likely have a more productive outcome.

Getting Clear on Your Why

Goals and vision are vital for growth in life, career, and relationships. Without them, we let life happen to us and give up our power and control to the winds of fate. What if I told you that you can have everything you need in life?

Now, don't get me wrong, obviously we can't control everything in life. Regaining your power has everything to do with understanding what you *can* and what you *cannot* control. And let me tell you one thing: the only thing you have control over is yourself. If you're unhappy about certain aspects of your life, it might be time to take back control. A good starting point is thinking about your vision and goals.

Sometimes used interchangeably, goals and vision are two separate, co-existing concepts. Your vision is your why. It provides direction and gives you the brush to paint the picture of a future you desire. Your vision is a powerful source of motivation. Once you've got a clear image of what your ideal future looks like, your goals are the practical steps that get you there.

Now, what do your goals and vision have to do with boundaries? Boundaries can serve as a powerful tool for achieving your goals and realizing your vision. Without clear boundaries, we move away from what we actually want and sometimes even forget what it was to begin with. Without a clear vision of what we want out of life, our need for boundaries might not be so apparent, since we are not prioritizing our own goals. We get so caught up in our daily lives and before we know it, years have gone by. People who never become fully aware of their true desires tend to feel generally dissatisfied in life without recognizing exactly why or how to fix it.

On the other hand, having clearly defined goals can make it easier to set boundaries. Once you've got your vision and the steps that will get you closer to it, you might find it easier to say 'no' to the people or commitments that do not serve you.

To help you on your way to imagining your vision you can use the exercise below. This is one of my favorite exercises because you can go all out on this one. I want to invite you to dream big and make it as specific as possible.

Exercise 1: *Visualize your Ideal Future*

Follow the next steps to the best of your abilities and you will maximize the potential effects that this practice has:

1. Treat this exercise like a meditation—sit in a calm environment, get comfortable, and start awakening your powerful imagination. You can even put on some meditation music if you want.
2. For this exercise, you can either focus on your whole life or a certain aspect of it (e.g., your relationships, work, money, health, etc.)
3. Close your eyes and take a few deep breaths until you feel your body and mind calming down. Focus on your breathing and *feel* the weight of gravity pulling you down into a deeper state of relaxation.
4. When you feel completely calm, I want you to start imagining your dream life (or an aspect of your dream life). What does this future look like? What are you doing? What do you feel like? What kind of a job do you have? How are your relationships? Who surrounds you? Who are you spending your time with? Where do you live? What does this environment look like? What do you look like? Try to imagine this future life in as much detail as possible. To solidify this, you can do this from both your point of view and an external point of view.
5. When you have a clear picture try to dig into your physical and emotional state. What does your body feel like? Any specific physical sensations? Do you feel proud? Giddy? Happy? Excited? Whatever you expect it to be, try to manufacture it in your state of visualization—truly *feel* that moment as if it's already happening.

6. Slowly bring your awareness back to the room around you and open your eyes.

When you're done with this exercise, I want you to write down your experience in detail. Look at the questions from the exercise and try to answer them. Hopefully, this was a beautiful experience that will stick with you for a long time. You can do this exercise as often as you want. Don't lose sight of the dream life you've imagined. Repeat this exercise often and focus on the aspects that make you happiest, honing in on your priorities. The more time you allow yourself to spend refining your vision, the easier it will be to determine what kind of goals you'll need to get there.

Exercise 2: Goal setting

Now that you have a clear vision I want you to pick an area of your dream life and start thinking about actionable goals to realize your vision.

The following questions can help you to make your goals more distinct and clearer:

- What is your goal? Describe it in one sentence.
- Why do you desire to achieve this goal? Are your intentions coming from a place of true fulfillment or rather gratification of vain desire?
- How do you believe you will feel and continue to live once your goal has been achieved?
- What are the biggest obstacles standing between you and this goal?
- Why haven't you started working toward this goal earlier? Be honest: Was it circumstance or something else (fear/intimidation/lack of discipline etc.)?
- Are you able to achieve this goal on your own or should you plan on seeking assistance from others?
- Is there anyone you look up to in terms of this goal? And why? Can you copy some of their habits/character traits?

- Do you have a relatively mapped-out idea of the steps you must take to achieve this goal?

Answering these questions not only grounds your belief that achieving this goal is truly valuable to your life, but also helps you to better communicate your desires and needs to achieve that goal.

If you ever feel yourself being pulled away from these goals by others, thinking of this exercise will help you to put out a more compelling case, giving the other person a better reason to attend to you. When you have a clear picture of what you want and don't want, it won't be as easy for people to derail you from it.

An Uncomfortable Truth

Annie Dillard once said: "How we spend our days is how we spend our lives." This quote has always resonated with me because it's such an obvious statement, but at the same time has a deeper meaning. As much as we'd like to, we can't change our lives in a day or a week. Change happens as a result of small adjustments on a day-to-day basis. Even the most driven people who fully embrace change frequently run into roadblocks that make their transformation far more challenging than originally expected.

We're often quite capable of envisioning our dream life and are actually quite good at setting goals. Who doesn't like to set a goal about earning more money? Or living a healthier life? The problem with keeping and achieving goals often has to do with facing one simple, but uncomfortable truth: if you want to change the world around you, it is *you* who needs to change. We would love to take control over our surroundings, circumstances, and other people, but the reality is that we can only control ourselves.

Obviously "changing yourself" is not as easy as it sounds. Believe me, this is my life's work. I know how hard it is to change yourself. But I'm seeing that it is possible, every single day, over and over again. With clearly defined goals and healthy boundaries in place, I have no doubt you can do the same.

Key Takeaways

- Boundaries are not about telling other people what to do, they're about validating your feelings and giving them space at the table
- By having a clear vision and setting practical goals we can create lasting change
- Boundaries help us to protect our vision and goals just as our goals help us to define clear boundaries
- Change happens in small increments and comes from within

Chapter 4
Why it's Hard to Set Boundaries

"When you say 'yes' to others, make sure you're not saying 'no' to yourself."

— *Paulo Coelho*

As social creatures, we have a primal need to belong to a community and form strong bonds of attachment with others. In the past, this was a matter of life or death. Early humans depended on collaboration, sharing knowledge, and pooling resources to grow in population. While the stakes are considerably lower today, imagine if you woke up tomorrow and your closest friend or romantic partner decided never speak to you again. This development would likely be devastating. You would feel crushed for losing someone that means so much to you. This need for closeness frequently causes us to disregard our personal boundaries and, in doing so, we end up dissatisfied.

The Lie of Selfishness

There's a reason why so many of us identify as people-pleasers. We are told that doing things for others is honorable and doing things for ourselves is not. The first half of that message is indeed correct—doing things for others is a good thing and expresses our compassion for them. However, for various reasons, many of us struggle with the feeling that being kind to ourselves is a form of vanity.

Let's make one thing clear: putting yourself first is *not* selfish. There's a saying I particularly like regarding this that goes "if you don't fill your gas tank, you can't carry passengers." You can't be expected to take care of others when you aren't taking care of yourself. I have many clients who work 60+ hours per week, still help their parents out around the house, and manage to raise a family while juggling their social life. Whenever we talk about self-care, they often tell me that it's just another item on their to-do list. One of my clients once said: "Taking a moment for myself feels more like a burden than something that makes me happy. I just don't have the time for it."

But when you are *always* attending to others, you are running on fumes. If your car runs out of gas, you don't keep slamming on the gas pedal, expecting it to move. You face the fact that you have to refuel it. Yet, you might struggle to apply the same strategy to yourself. You could be exhausted before you even step out of bed, yet if your phone rings with an urgent request from a coworker, your mouth will be saying 'sure' before your head has even realized what it signed up for.

I'll reiterate this: by saying 'no' to others, you're saying 'yes' to yourself. But how often do you actually do that? Taking some time for yourself simply ensures that you give the same amount of care that you show to others to yourself. Anyone who doesn't let you do that is not a friend of yours and they will not be getting your best.

Selfishness is when someone is concerned solely with their own happiness and well-being and does not care about others. Kindly telling someone you would prefer to stay in and recharge rather than help them with a project on your day off is far from selfish. It's time to change the narrative and take back your power to determine the things you dedicate your time and energy to.

In my journey to set healthy boundaries I learned a very important lesson. The only people who reacted negatively when I finally set firm boundaries were the ones who had benefited from trampling over mine for many years. As I'm sure many others can relate, one of my strongest barriers was the idea that people close to me would find my new determination selfish or rude. I knew this feeling came from a place of insecurity, but I couldn't shake it off until I understood one important concept. It suddenly clicked. If people around me are angry because I can't commit to helping them at the expense of my own obligations, they don't respect my time. Or if they are hurt by the fact I can no longer lend them money because I need it myself, they do not respect my financial well-being.

The People-Pleasing Habit

In extreme cases, people-pleasing can be associated with a personality trait known as *sociotropy,* or being overly concerned with pleasing others to sustain relationships. Someone with sociotropy will overvalue social acceptance to the point they struggle with the possibility of a negative outcome. They feel as if they are obligated to change their approach to the relationship or put in a greater effort to produce a positive final result. If their partner comes home in a bad mood due to something that occurred at work, simply comforting their partner would not feel like enough. They would have to do anything in their power to make their partner feel better and try to 'fix' the situation. This type of person will go to extreme lengths to make their partner feel better and are so fixated on solving the problem they may become misguided in their approach. But, thinking that their partner's mood at the end of the day is entirely dependent on their actions is not only damaging but completely unrealistic.

A person with sociotropy also tends to place the well-being of others above their own happiness and independence. They will sacrifice their autonomy, all of their time, a lot of their money, and other aspects of their independence in an attempt to maintain closeness in the relationship. Consequently, they are deeply affected by a relationship ending or even some conflict arising within it. It's probably obvious at this point that someone with sociotropy struggles to lead a happy life for themselves and often gives up self-respect and their independence for something that is ultimately far beyond their control.

Not nearly all people-pleasers suffer from sociotropy, though it bears mentioning as the extremes to which people-pleasing can go. For example, one of the biggest characteristics of a people-pleaser is putting someone else's happiness above your own well-being. People-pleasing is a harmful trait and many of us find ourselves somewhere on the spectrum.

So, *why* is it that people-pleasing is so common? In reality, there are many possible causes, including:

- Trauma, especially from childhood or past relationships
- Being upheld to unrealistically high expectations by your family and feeling as if you were never enough
- Only being granted attention and care from those around you if you do as they say
- Feeling unseen by those you care about as if your needs are not as important as their expectations
- You want the person you are trying to please to be indebted to you
- You are afraid of the relationship ending if you don't adhere to the other person's every requirement

People-pleasing is inherently contradictory to the concept of setting boundaries. Why? Because the former is done solely for your counterpart and the latter is done for *your* benefit. People who cannot kick their people-pleasing habit will have a hard time motivating themselves to set boundaries and accepting the possibility of introducing conflict to a relationship.

Are you a people-pleaser? Even if you say no, perhaps you might still exhibit some aspects of this habit. Here are 10 signs that you might be somewhat of a people-pleaser (Morin, 2017):

1. You pretend to agree with people's opinions even if you do not.
2. You feel a strong sense of responsibility for other people's emotions.
3. You apologize too often—almost habitually.
4. You feel exhausted with your schedule, especially if it is filled to the brim with activities you feel pressured to join in on but do not enjoy.
5. You struggle to say 'no'.
6. You can't handle it when someone close to you is upset with you.
7. You often take on the personalities or behaviors of those around you.
8. You seek constant validation and reassurance to believe someone likes you.
9. You would do anything to prevent a conflict with someone.
10. You keep it to yourself if you are upset and suppress negative emotions

Being a people-pleaser is nothing to be ashamed of. The concept of social conformity affects all of us and has been the topic of study for many sociologists and psychologists for decades.

As has been a recurring theme throughout the past several chapters, we are relatively easily influenced by those around us. In fact, we are affected even by those who might be physically distant, yet their influence reigns over us.

The process of kicking the pesky habit of people-pleasing is not an overnight change. It is a process of reprogramming not only how you view others, but how you view yourself as well. Distancing yourself from some people-pleasing habits will have some overlap with a technique that is familiar to us all: setting goals and prioritizing your own life. When we set goals for ourselves and visualize a desirable outcome, we remind ourselves that the happiness of those around us is not the defining component of *our* happiness. When we start prioritizing ourselves, we are recovering from that habit of only ever pleasing others. Furthermore, it opens our eyes to the undeniable fact that we cannot possibly build up to our future achievements if we spend our present solely worried about others who do not reciprocate this energy. Once we are clear on our desires, we can fully commit to them by being radically honest. Yes, keeping them to ourselves protects us from possible conflict in the short run, but by always being truthful we will reap the benefits in the mid to long-term.

Other than reminding ourselves of our desires and goals, we could also (Cherry, 2021):

- Start small. When training to be able to stand up for ourselves, we can start practicing on things that hold little significance. For example, politely say no to a small request that will barely affect the other person; or you could voice your opinion to someone even if they have a different point of view on something. You could even try to say 'no' through a text or email and then work your way up to telling people 'no' in person.
- Practice positive and uplifting self-talk. We are constantly talking to ourselves and about ourselves, even if we don't notice or admit it. What we say is very important. So, start watching and noticing your thoughts about yourself: Do you put yourself down? Do you justify the poor treatment you are offered by others? If so, start shifting your self-talk from "I owe this person my time" to something like "I am owed the autonomy to spend my time how I wish."
- Don't immediately say yes to requests. If someone asks you for yet another favor, don't say yes right at that moment, even if you have to bite your tongue. Instead, say something along the lines of "I'm not sure at the moment, but let me get back to you." By saying this, you are not only preventing yourself from agreeing to something prematurely but it might be easier for

you to decline their favor when you're not in the heat of the moment. Before you give them your final answer, you have the time to evaluate whether you can (or should) commit to it.

- Assess if the person is asking or expecting too much of you. If someone is asking you for something, stop and think about their pattern of behavior. How often do they ask you for something? Is their request reasonable? Are they someone who reciprocates your efforts and helps you out from time to time? Will they have a negative or nasty reaction if you were to decline (i.e. do they feel entitled to your time and efforts)?
- Remind yourself that relationships of all kinds require reciprocation. If a friend, for example, only takes and takes without giving you anything back, they are flat-out being a bad friend. Perhaps talking to them and setting some boundaries will help them adjust their behavior.

When you are just starting out in your recovery from people-pleasing, you might be tempted to cut some corners to make the process easier for yourself and I don't blame you! There is no shame in this—as long as you are trying and making some progress, you are already taking one step toward the new you.

A lot of people find that they need to justify all of their answers to a fault. This can look like a rambling, detailed explanation as to *why* they are saying no to a particular request. I understand why this might be tempting for someone who is used to always saying yes, but unfortunately, when you do this, you continue to invalidate yourself. By overly explaining why you are declining a request, you communicate that you can't justify your reasons for doing so. The bottom line is that we do not need to justify our answer to someone's request. We can just say no, simply because we feel like it.

Clouded by Society

Going back to our human need for belonging, social norms and expectations weigh heavily on how we view boundaries and the values we prioritize. Although we are living through a period of rapid social change, we continue to be strongly encouraged to behave and relate to others in specific ways that are rewarded by the society we belong to. Therefore it is important to examine how susceptible we are to limiting our individuality in an effort to fit in.

My grandmother was a great example of someone who was successfully convinced by society that she owed it all to my grandfather. Now, to be clear, he was a great man, but the norms society instilled in both of their heads hovered over them their entire lives, well into the 21st century. She moved in with him straight from her parent's house and became a stay-at-home wife the moment they got married. Throughout my entire childhood, she told me all about the 'lovely' things she got to do while at home. She said she was perfectly satisfied taking care of the house and turning it into a home. Eventually, they had four children, and her time became occupied with them. My grandfather worked and was the traditional breadwinner.

As I became older, I started to see the cracks in their stories and the doubt behind their smiles. When I was in my twenties, my grandmother and I had a heartfelt conversation in which she encouraged me to take advantage of all the opportunities presented to me while expressing some regrets from her past. She told me about her passion for science and her fascination with the stars. Deep down she wanted to be an astronomer but never even got the chance to learn about such a subject. It was the only time she ever shared this truth about her desires, and it pained me to hear her lament the missed opportunities in her life. Shortly after she passed away, my grandfather also spoke more openly about how the expectations of his time had influenced his choices. He was always such a powerful, artsy inspiration in my life. He was a fantastic painter when he eventually retired and even started learning the piano when he was 68 years old. He too had wanted to live a life that was different from the one he had led. One filled with art instead of machines in an industrial factory. I believe they were genuinely happy at the end of their lives, but it was striking to hear them both refer to society-induced limitations being among their life's greatest regrets.

It's easier said than done to live a life untethered by others and unchained from social constructs. But seeing how our independent desires are formed and influenced by culture and society is a good first step.

Key Takeaways

- While helping others is certainly a good trait, it becomes draining if others' needs become prioritized over your own.
- Sociotropy is a trait closely related to people-pleasing, causing someone to be overly invested in making others happy.
- People-pleasing causes someone to avoid conflict and can prevent them from setting boundaries.
- Society has a strong influence over our views of relationships and our role in them.

Chapter 5
Unearthing Your Self-Worth

Strong people have a strong sense of self-worth and self-awareness;
they don't need the approval of others.

— *Roy T. Bennett*

There is a reason why so much material regarding boundary-setting is directly correlated with how confident we are in ourselves. Think of someone confident, do you imagine them letting others walk all over them? Do they agree to things they don't want to do and regret not doing what they wanted? Or are they able to casually say 'no' in a way that makes others respect their response without demanding an explanation?

One fool-proof way of checking if someone respects you or not is how they respond to your 'no.' If they poke holes in it, demand to know every little detail about why you are choosing to say 'no', or attempt to turn your 'no' into a 'yes', it could indicate they don't respect you or your time. Being made to feel obligated to justify your answer is an indication the other person won't respect your answer unless their ego deems it valid. To change this, we need to learn how to stand our ground. To confront another's *ego*, we benefit from understanding ourselves and augmenting our confidence and self-esteem.

It is important to note the key difference between ego and self-esteem. Self-esteem is one's *confidence* in their own capabilities and skills. It comes from within. Ego, however, is the *opinion* a person has of themself and is based on external validation. Ego says more about how important one feels around others whereas self-esteem is a measure of self-respect.

Let's take a difficult job interview as an example. A person with low self-esteem will be bombarded with doubt leading up to the said interview. They might procrastinate out of fear, feel extremely anxious, or even give up before trying. Someone with healthy self-esteem is excited about such a challenge with a potential reward. They will approach it differently: They will grab the tools and resources they need and start preparing to give their best. They believe they deserve to give this interview their best shot because they have what it takes to get the job.

A person with an inflated ego could be presumptuous and go into the interview assuming they will automatically move to the next round simply because they deserve this job. An inflated sense of self-importance and entitlement guides this belief rather than authentic confidence in their abilities or self-worth. They might not even prepare for the interview or plan to outsmart or manipulate the interviewers.

A particularly egotistical person will likely set unequal boundaries. They will set boundaries that only benefit them while exploiting others. Oftentimes, these attempts are manipulative in nature. For example, they might say "I feel neglected if you don't spend every free night with me. I should be your priority and I feel like you spending time with your friends is disrespectful to our relationship." Hopefully, this doesn't sound familiar to any of you, but it happens more often than one might think.

Oddly enough, society tends to reward ego-fueled achievements, so we're destined to have our boundaries challenged by a few inflated egos throughout our journey of life. The best way to handle toxic egotistical behavior rests in a defined sense of self-worth. We'll be discussing techniques to examine our self-esteem in the next section. These exercises should make you more comfortable in your power, opening the door to becoming more assertive when needed.

Self-Worth Theory

The way people view themselves is such a complex thing to understand, there are entire branches of psychology dedicated to figuring it out. Isn't that ironic? One of the hardest things for us to understand in life is ourselves. The self-worth theory is a psychological theory that states the ultimate goal in people's lives is finding self-worth through self-acceptance and achievement (Ackerman, 2018).

The theory goes on to describe that there are four key components that make up the self-worth model:

- Ability
- Effort
- Performance
- Self-worth

The first three bullet points interplay with each other to make up your self-worth. If you have strong abilities and put in enough effort, your performance will likely be exceptional. When your performance is good, your self-worth will be as well.

While this theory is a decent representation of many people's mentalities, it doesn't cover the entire truth. Yes, our achievements play a massive role in the way we view ourselves and how much we think we are worth. However, if our self-worth is *entirely* rooted in achievement, we risk losing it at the first sign of failure. Life isn't linear—we will have good days, bad days, great days, and awful days. If we attach our worth to these ever-changing conditions, we give up stability.

The Determinants

Here are some good questions to ask yourself: What makes you feel good about yourself? What makes you feel bad about yourself? And what factors can you identify that determine how much worth you see in yourself?

Everyone's answers will be different, but research has found that some factors tend to generally overlap. Those commonly mentioned factors can be categorized as follows (Ackerman, 2018):

- Appearance
- Net worth and finances
- Our social network
- Our career success
- Achievements

Getting into college, being accepted for a job or a promotion, trying to appear a certain way to others; our lives are filled with competition. It's a universal trait for us to feel good when we manage to do something a little better than others. It proves our ability to meaningfully contribute to society, nurturing our need for belonging. This is naturally ingrained in most of us, but it doesn't necessarily serve us in regard to our self-worth. We have to learn that our worth runs so much deeper than our achievements. You are worthy simply because you exist, nothing more. Self-worth should come from a place of unconditional love. Instead of getting caught up in chasing money, status and popularity we should work on identifying and challenging our critical inner voice. Fully commit to treating yourself with kindness, tolerance, generosity, and compassion.

Seeing Neutrality

My niece is someone I'm very close to in this life. She's a wonderful young woman, and she and I get along very well. In her teens, however, she began to struggle with her self-esteem and adopted quite an unhealthy self-image. She tried for years to find her confidence but her high school years were, simply put, hellish.

She focused on every superficial quality imaginable. Her lack of wealth was embarrassing, her body was ugly and she felt inferior to her peers.

My niece is a go-getter and she set out to tackle these perceived short-comings with a vengeance. I had to give it to her, even if I disagreed with her approach. She was able to achieve the appearance of a lifestyle she wanted via social media channels and she felt more confident because of it. She had confronted her insecurities by achieving an image of superiority - being the best, more beautiful, more successful than her peers. But as soon as she got negative feedback, the fragility of her meticulously built house of cards became apparent and her self-esteem took a nosedive.

So I introduced her to a new approach: the rule of neutrality. The rule of neutrality is simply the concept of seeing yourself as neither good nor bad. If you hate the way you look today, you don't have to convince yourself you're beautiful. Instead, start telling yourself you're simply in a body—its beauty is subjective, and you have no obligation to see yourself as a walking god or goddess; your body's beauty or lack thereof is not a determinant of your worth. No one of us is truly, objectively, more beautiful than anyone else.

I told my niece to apply this to all the areas she lacked confidence in. She doesn't need to think she's a genius, but she also doesn't need to tell herself she is unintelligent; she doesn't have to think her clothes are runway-worthy, but she shouldn't see them as rags either. After all, these are egotistical desires and her authentic worth was unattached to any of these aspects. It wasn't easy and it took her some years, but eventually, she became comfortable with neutrality. She was able to look at other girls and say "yes, she has fashionable clothes and a body that wears them well, but I wear my style in my own way."

It was only after she accepted the fact that there will always be something or someone better, she started to transition into a more confident woman. Her clothes served their purpose, her body was doing everything it was supposed to, the amount of money she had was nobody's business. With the gratitude she found through the rule of neutrality, she was able to shift toward a more positive mindset and higher self-esteem.

I would invite you to try it yourself. Treat neutrality as the foundation on which your future confidence and self-esteem will be based. See yourself as neutral: you are simply you. Feel the balance within your life, push away the superficial labels. Yes, there are aspects of your life that can be improved but that is no reason to hate them as they are right now.

Understanding Potential

As you probably noticed in my earlier example about self-esteem versus ego, someone with healthy self-esteem holds confidence in the things they believe they are capable of. Yes, their self-esteem is probably based on their successes from the past, but even with the fluctuations of successes and failures, they continue to believe that they will be just as capable to meet future challenges.

People who have good self-esteem generally have at least a basic sense of their skills and what they are good at or can become good at. Now, to truly know your capabilities and inclinations you might require some in-depth soul-searching but getting to know yourself is worth it in the long run.

"But, what if I'm not particularly good at anything? Will I not be able to develop my self-esteem?" A valid question considering what we just discussed, but the answer is a resounding 'yes'. First of all, there is always some area in your life where you excel. Perhaps you don't place a particularly high value on that skill or talent, but I refuse to believe there is anyone on this earth that does not excel in one thing or another, no matter how trivial it may seem. Another important thing to understand is that our abilities are dynamic, not static. This is part of the larger concept of a growth mindset versus a fixed mindset. In short, a growth mindset is when a person believes they can become good at new things, learn additional skills, and improve upon existing ones. A fixed mindset is at the opposite end of that spectrum and is present when a person thinks their skills are determined by chance and they are not capable of changing their potency.

You don't have to be a wunderkind at something to develop your self-esteem. However, you must strive toward something and believe in yourself. Allow yourself to acknowledge the areas where you excel. Try to see the skills or character traits you possess as your small contribution to the world around you. Give that contribution some validation and take ownership. There are billions of us on this earth and we all have but a tiny part to play in the human story. Once you're able to accept that you possess unique skills or character traits that make your contribution unique, it is easier to believe you are worthy of achieving greater things. Accept what you're already good at, validate the notion that you are capable of achieving great things and let that fuel your ability to develop new skills as well.

If this all sounds a bit ambiguous, try doing the visualization technique we went over in chapter 3. Identify a goal that takes you just one step closer to a vision that makes you happiest, and go for it.

Accepting Compliments

Whenever I mention that accepting compliments is directly tied to a person's ability to set solid boundaries, people get confused. Soon, the correlation will make sense.

There are four common reasons why a person might struggle to accept the compliments they are given (Morin, 2016):

1. **Low self-esteem.** Hey, we just talked about that! Low self-esteem isn't just not believing in yourself, but it's also a refusal to accept that *others* can believe in you. In other words, you have so little faith in yourself that you can't fathom the idea that others have faith in you. For example, if you think you have awful taste in style, it is almost jarring to hear someone compliment your outfit—so much so that it is unbelievable to you.

2. **Different self-image.** Even without low self-esteem, we struggle to wrap our heads around the fact that people view us differently from how we view ourselves. Furthermore, each person views us a bit differently than the next. This inconsistency between how we are told we are viewed compared to how we view ourselves is often referred to as cognitive dissonance. When a person compliments us on a trait we perceive as a flaw, we will struggle to accept it. A compliment like that will make you either reconsider your self-image or question the other person's honesty.

3. **Your bar is lower than theirs.** Oftentimes, people who cannot accept compliments simply diminish their successes and skills. They tend to shy away from others' expectations if they appear to be too big. To someone like this, a compliment like "you're such a hard worker," might trigger anxiety because they don't want to disappoint when they don't live up to their expectations.

4. **You want to stay humble.** This is a trait that is shared by most people. Even those that don't struggle to accept compliments do struggle with finding a balanced response to them. If we were to agree with the person giving a compliment, we often view ourselves as coming off cocky. "You are such a talented student," is hard to follow with "yes, I agree." So, to avoid reacting in a potentially arrogant manner, we often resort to disagreeing with the compliment altogether. Instead, the proper solution to this problem would be to thank the person for the compliment without agreeing or disagreeing with it.

In full transparency, accepting compliments will continue to be difficult as long as your self-esteem and self-worth are below healthy levels. Therefore, you must start applying the rule of neutrality, increase your self-esteem, and then start to accept compliments as they were meant to be received.

The ability to accept compliments is important for someone trying to set boundaries. Accepting a compliment and forming a boundary are both manifestations of how we interact with others and allow outsiders to view us. When we properly acknowledge a compliment and receive it well, we are allowing that person to view us in a positive light and accept that we are worthy of praise. When communicating our boundaries, we are enforcing a similar concept. We are laying out a framework that governs how a person can interact with us while acknowledging that our autonomy, time, and mental health is worth preserving. One action is more passive—receiving a compliment—and the other occurs only through applied action—setting boundaries.

If we don't allow ourselves to accept compliments, we are furthering the idea that we mean very little to others. When we start believing compliments and accepting them, we are solidifying the idea that we are worthy of respect. The more we communicate to the world that we are worthy of respect, the easier it becomes to set healthy boundaries.

Direct Action

The way we view ourselves largely shapes the type of life we have. Perspective is everything, truly. It's easier said than done, but a simple shift in mindset is sometimes enough to get a glimpse of the light at the end of the tunnel. There are people who are naturally predisposed toward a more optimistic outlook on their life just as there are people who tend to view things in a more negative light. In some instances, perspective can be heavily skewed by common mental health issues such as depression or anxiety, but more often it is simply a case of a nasty habit.

Are there times when you feel negativity taking over in your own thoughts? Here's a list of a few things you can start doing today to become a more positive person. Seeing the world and your life in a more positive light can work wonders on improving your self-esteem:

- **Practice being more grateful.** Easy, right? Well, I'm giving you some homework. Take out a journal and list five things you are grateful for today. Make it a new habit to do this every day. By bringing our conscious attention to what we are happy to have in our lives, we balance out our perception of the negatives. You can even start improving your self-esteem by writing things about yourself you are grateful for—even the smallest things will do!

- **Evaluate your skills.** There's good and bad in everything. So, be as objective as possible and write a list of things you believe yourself to be good at and a list of things you would describe as your weak points. Now, look at the list of weaknesses: Is there anything on there that you would like to be good at? Thanks to the human's ability to fluidly change our abilities, you can be! You don't have to be perfect, but you can get a jolt of positivity by attempting something you may have written off as a weakness and improving that skill even slightly.

- **Surround yourself with good people.** If you are someone who is developing a new version of yourself and wants to find new passions in life, you will need the right people surrounding you for support. If someone drains you of your positivity— through constant negative reassurance—they are probably holding you back. Try to surround yourself with people who uplift and inspire you, as well as those who make the effort to create positive change within their own lives.

- **Don't feel guilty about your happiness.** Start prioritizing your joy. You can do this by putting time aside every day to do something you love just for you. Once you start prioritizing your happiness you will see the critical need for boundaries. So, go out there and try out that restaurant you've been eyeing for the past year, go on a trip with your best friend, or start learning a new language!

As you start improving other areas of your life, you will begin to realize the importance of having firm boundaries. You might even start noticing just how much you used to do for others while putting your own happiness on the back burner.

Key Takeaways

- Ego is about the blind belief that one is better than another, while self-esteem is about knowing one's true worth.
- The self-worth theory describes four key components that dictate how we value ourselves: ability, effort, performance, and self-worth.
- If you are insecure about yourself, working toward a place of neutrality is the first step in gaining more confidence.
- Developing good self-esteem has to do with believing in your ability to conquer adversity—don't shy away from a challenge.
- Accepting compliments is important for your sense of self-worth and becoming comfortable with others acknowledging it.
- Improving surrounding areas of your life will directly boost your self-esteem as your overall satisfaction increases.

Chapter 6
Setting Boundaries Starts with You

Healing may not be so much about getting better, as about letting go of everything that isn't you—all of the expectations, all of the beliefs—and becoming who you are.

— *Rachel Naomi Remen*

As you might have grasped by now, setting boundaries has more to do with ourselves than others. By understanding ourselves and facing our own demons, we become better at setting healthy boundaries.

Reasonable boundaries come from a place of respect, value, and love. Manifestations of deep insecurities, on the other hand, are nagging feelings that make you feel unworthy without anyone else's wrongdoing. These little pesky insecurities get the best of us, which is why every once in a while, we'll feel like we're getting eaten up with an emotion we don't want to feel in the first place. To create healthier boundaries, we first need to figure out whether our needs are representative of something *we* need to work on or if it's something that concerns others.

Shadow Work and You

Shadow work, a practice developed by the famed Swiss psychologist Carl Jung, is a method that helps one answer questions they are often afraid of asking themself, thus freeing them from their secrets and allowing them to identify the boundaries they would want to set. The great thing about shadow work is that it is highly customizable and you can practice it for years without reaching the end of its usefulness. Getting to know yourself is a never-ending process.

According to Jung, each one of us has a persona. Think of this as the mask we wear to project a certain image of ourselves to the outside world. We also each have a shadow side. Our shadow tends to be the opposite of this conscious personality and can be instinctive and irrational.

Shadow work is meant to unveil what is beneath that mask, specifically the parts of ourselves that we tend to reject and generally cover-up. For example, having aggressive or mean tendencies would certainly be something that the persona of a hyper-agreeable person would try to mask, as they don't want to be associated with such attributes.

These darker parts of ourselves can be quite frightening to acknowledge and confront—even admitting to ourselves that we have them can be difficult to get through. However, by giving these darker parts of yourself attention through shadow work, you will be taking away their power and getting in touch with what you actually want to express.

To get started with some basic shadow work, sit down in a calm environment with a journal and a pen, and start answering these questions:

- Do I feel like I treat myself with kindness and respect—the same way I should expect someone else to treat me?
- Do I often allow others to treat me with less kindness and respect than I deserve?
- What are some examples of healthy and happy relationships that I've witnessed? What do I like about them?

- What are some examples of unhealthy relationships that I've witnessed? What were the issues?
- How easy is it for me to see someone for exactly who they are without unrealistically idolizing them?
- Do I struggle to confront a person when they have done me wrong? If so, what feelings do I experience at the thought of confronting them?
- What do I feel when my best friend seems to be spending more time with their other friends than with me? What is/would be my reaction?
- How easily do I get jealous in romantic relationships?
- Can I easily and neutrally accept the fact that my romantic partner has been with other people before me?
- Can I easily and neutrally accept the fact that my ex is with other people following our breakup?
- Am I holding on to any feelings or resentment from my past relationships? If so, what are they, and why is it so difficult for me to let go of them?
- Do I truly believe I am being realistic when it comes to wanting a relationship? Do I expect them to be perfect and solve all of my problems or do I understand that relationships are never perfect and require work from both parties?

It is important to understand that your shadow is not a shortcoming or a mistake, but rather an inherent part of who you are. Ultimately, the goal of shadow work is to gain self-awareness. It enables you to recognize the various parts of yourself. When we start to embrace these darker parts of ourselves, we obtain control and can start showing up as our authentic selves.

Setting Boundaries with Yourself

We tend to think of boundaries as a way to communicate our limits with others, but we also need to consider the boundaries we set for ourselves. These boundaries enable us to uphold a certain lifestyle, maintain stability, and stay healthy.

Everyone has their own set of boundaries. The limits you set for yourself might be very different from others, but let's take a look at some examples to give you a general idea of what your boundaries could be:

- Sticking to a budget
- Not answering work emails on the weekends
- No phones or TV allowed in the bedroom
- Not using social media when you're bored
- Avoiding unhealthy foods
- Having no more than 2 cups of coffee a day
- Not drinking alcohol during the week

The majority of us struggle to keep certain self-imposed limits. We all understand the benefits of discipline and limitations, yet it can be challenging to follow them. However, when we change our perception and start to understand these boundaries as a means to achieve our goals, perhaps we can view them in a better light. You're not depriving yourself from having a bag of Doritos, you're working on becoming healthier. You're not missing out on a chance to let loose with friends, you are prioritizing rest. Boundaries around the things that interfere with our goals allow us to ultimately live a happier life.

Your Inner Child

Some of us must use self-imposed boundaries as a means to *re-parent* ourselves. That's to say, we are providing ourselves with the limits that might have been lacking in our childhood.

As children, we are subject to whatever conditions our parents or guardians put us in. We have very little say in the matter as we are too young to be independent. We are completely reliant on those who hold the responsibility to take care of us.

If you were lucky, your parents had healthy boundaries themselves and taught you to internalize the ability to set healthy boundaries as well. But in reality, most childhoods are flawed in some way or another. I like to believe that every parent does the best they can for their children, but this is of course limited by a parent's own abilities and shaped by their life experience. We pass down the things we know - the good, the bad and the ugly.

Many times, we are well aware of our limits and know when we don't agree with something. However, we struggle to say 'no' in these situations and often end up agreeing anyway; we know we should've declined and may even beat ourselves up for not having the courage to do so. Such compliance and fear of conflict is often rooted in deeper-set issues that stem from the way we were treated as children.

Our primary caretaker might've been too busy at work to provide us with the quality time we needed, might've been too stressed to be emotionally present, or might have even been struggling with a mental health issue that rendered them emotionally unpredictable. A plethora of possibilities can stunt our development and instill the need for constant reassurance, fear of abandonment, excessive people-pleasing, trust issues, and an inability to set boundaries.

Let's explore some of the common childhood conditions that produce emotional difficulties into adulthood. These are important factors to evaluate in your own life to recognize the potential root of your struggles:

1. Your guardian was often too busy to spend adequate time with you. If as a child you were always looking to spend even a sliver of time with a parent you loved but didn't get to see enough, you might develop an overly demanding emotional attachment to others. You could struggle with the idea of going long periods of time without seeing someone you care about. This could actually cause *them* to set a boundary with you if they felt it was a bit overbearing. You may, on the other hand, need boundaries that protect your need to feel cared for.
2. Your guardian only complimented you and showed you affection when you achieved something. It makes sense for those who are in charge of our growing process to want us to

succeed. However, many parents take this to the extreme; they treat their love as a sort of reward. Therefore, it was only expressed to their child if they had achieved something. This form of parenting is harmful and reinforces the idea in a child's mind that they must be successful in areas predetermined by their parents in order to deserve to receive love. This doesn't take into account the differences in people's capabilities, interests, and emotional needs. In adulthood this often manifests as over-achievement, doing things solely for the approval of others, and valuing the opinions of others more than your own.

3. Your guardians were not happy with you unless you were following the trajectory they created for you. I've seen many overbearing parents like this; they live vicariously through their children and cannot accept them as individuals that are separate from them. They expect their children to do just as well in school, love the same things, and do well in the areas they have (or haven't!) excelled at. When they grow up, these kids might not only have a lost sense of identity, but they may succumb to extreme people-pleasing because it's the only way to make sure they receive the love they seek.

4. Your guardians often compared you to others or belittled your individuality. Demanding autonomy is difficult. Saying no is also very difficult. If these skills aren't given the space to blossom in one's early stages of life, they become particularly hard to develop. If a child was often made to feel inferior or as if they could never be as good as others, they struggle to develop the confidence and self-esteem to believe that their 'no' holds value.

Parents and teachers are our first examples of what it means to be an adult. In a perfect world, they demonstrate good conflict resolution, clear communication, mutual respect, and care for their peers. But without active parenting, many lessons can simply glide over a child's head. Adults who grew up in such childhood conditions might be unable to rely on or trust others and therefore set either overly aggressive boundaries or become completely reliant on others.

Healing Childhood Wounds

Difficulties from a person's childhood will remain present for a lifetime. The things ingrained in us during our formative years will always be with us, and the qualities that prevent us from engaging with the world in healthy ways must be addressed. We are presented with two options: to suppress our childhood pain and allow it to continue to poison our lives, or take some difficult steps to confront that pain, make peace with it and put it in its place so we can grow beyond our past.

The fear of abandonment, fear of rejection, difficulty trusting others, co-dependence, and similar issues interfere with our ability to form strong bonds and nurture healthy relationships. By addressing these things, you make it easier for yourself to live the life you desire.

Therapist Andrea Brandt (2018) outlines a step-by-step method of starting to process your childhood wounds:

1. **Connect with yourself.** Begin this process by grounding yourself, your body, and your mind. Simply sit quietly in a comfortable position and bring attention to all of your bodily sensations. Close your eyes, take some deep breaths, and allow your body and mind to be present in that moment. Center yourself by feeling a flow of energy move from the bottom of your spine, into the ground, and all the way into the layers of the earth.

2. **Recall an emotional reaction.** Now that you are present with yourself, think back to a recent incident that produced undesirable feelings within you. It could be when you felt disrespected by a coworker, jealous of your partner, resentful toward a friend, or disappointed by a family member—anything that made you feel unpleasant. Review what led up to you being upset and what about it made you feel the way you did. Notice the details and

visualize yourself living through that moment all over again. When you successfully do this to the point of bringing those emotions back up to the surface, proceed to the following step.

3. **Sense the emotions.** As the emotions start to become stronger, allow yourself to sense them throughout your entire body. Try to pinpoint any physical responses to these emotions that you might be experiencing—tingling, tension, pain, etc. As you scan your body and find these physical sensations, try to carefully describe them to yourself. As soon as you feel that you've identified and described all appropriate physical sensations, you can carry on.

4. **Attach a name to it.** Now, try to identify what each emotion is. If you felt your arms tense up, is this because of anger or frustration? Is the tingling sensation in your chest jealousy? Is your breath feeling shallow because you feel anxious or as if you are in danger? Try to name the emotions that you feel associated with your body's reactions. Go as far as you can to get to the core emotion. For example, "I am disappointed in my friend because she forgot to call me on my birthday" could mean "I am sad because it appears she doesn't care about me".

5. **Assess the situation.** Is this emotion valid? Following the previous example, you could ask yourself: Was it my friend's intention to hurt me? Does she really not care about me? Or are there other possible reasons why she might have forgotten my birthday? Quite possibly you can think of a million possibilities why she forgot to call you. But why do you think you went straight for the worst possible reason? It is worth noticing here that we often don't respond to a situation, we respond to our interpretation of what's happening. Most likely, this situation triggered something in you that is rooted in something that happened to you in the past.

6. **Comfort yourself.** It's difficult to love someone that causes us pain, but what if that someone is yourself? We might, at a deep level, believe we're not worthy of love and respect. Recognize that whatever you have gone through in the past needs acknowledgment and validation. You needed and deserved love

at that moment. The beautiful thing is that you can give it to yourself at this very moment. Love yourself even with all the difficult emotions that you experience.

7. **Embrace all of it.** These feelings are there for a reason and they aren't going to go away instantly. So, sit with them and allow yourself to feel them in full. Don't lie to yourself about not feeling them, don't judge them, and don't minimize how strongly you feel them—just feel them from a point of neutrality. This might take a while, but only move on to the next step when you feel like you've truly felt all of your emotions in full and given them validation.

8. **Learn the lessons.** The emotions you experience are part of a bigger picture; They are telling you something you need to change about either your environment and your life or about yourself. For this step, dig deep within those emotions and try identifying other circumstances that triggered you to feel this way. Notice any patterns, and if you do see similarities, try to get to the very root of the problem and figure out why these situations have such an impact on you.

Dealing with our childhood wounds can be an intimidating and vulnerable task, but we have to remind ourselves that it all lies in the past. We are adults now and are no longer limited by our young age or the need to follow others' authority. We can heal the parts of ourselves that were damaged when we were younger and can learn to stand up for ourselves as adults.

Key Takeaways

- Setting boundaries healthy requires self-reflection.
- Shadow work uses powerful questions to allow you to learn your own needs and assess your satisfaction in your relationships.
- We need to change our perspective on the boundaries we set with ourselves - they are there to help us achieve what we authentically want.

- The way we were treated by adults when we were children can influence how we treat others in adulthood.
- Wounds that are left throughout our childhood manifest in conflict and insecurities when we become adults—it is necessary to acknowledge them and heal them.

Chapter 7
How to Go About It

"Daring to set boundaries is about having the courage to love ourselves even when we risk disappointing others."

— *Brené Brown*

We've figured out the what and the why, but now it is time to get into the *how*. Practically, we have yet to test our theory. Getting around to setting the boundaries can take a while as it can be nerve-wracking, as this is the point where we break out from the comfort zone.

Regaining Your Individuality

First, let's get one thing straight: your life is yours to live. Sometimes, even the hardest of decisions may be necessary for you to preserve your well-being. Once you start valuing your individuality, you will start realizing your worth.

In the previous chapters, we talked about the difference between rational boundaries and emotionally-clouded boundaries. Ideally, your boundaries should genuinely represent your value system and apply those values to the relationships in which you participate. When your boundaries come from a healthy place, then you need not worry about situations that expose your misalignment with others. For example, if you are the type to diligently structure your schedule, you shouldn't feel bad about saying 'no' to a last-minute invitation or request for your help.

Maintaining your individuality in relationships is crucial for your health. In order to do so we must uphold three things: independence, autonomy, and 0ur own point of view (Firestone, 2018). We should have a good sense of who we are inside and outside of all our relationships—you shouldn't be defined by another person's expectations of you.

Here are a few pointers on how to strengthen your sense of self to prevent it from being mangled by others:

- Try to make more personal decisions without heavily relying on the input of others. If you're wondering whether you should quit your job and find a new career path, for example, make the decision based on your own perception. Yes, of course you could ask others for their input, but don't overly rely on their opinions. After all, everyone will present you with a different perspective. Trust yourself because you are the only person with all the facts of the matter, and you alone are capable of knowing what you truly want.
- You do the things you choose not to satisfy others, but because they fulfill you. It can be difficult to completely detach yourself from other people's feelings, but you can always start small. Pick up a hobby that you've always wanted to try even if you think your peers will find it lame. Satisfy your own needs without being responsible for their feelings about it. If *you* enjoy something, you deserve to spend your time doing it.
- You are at peace with your own feelings. If you are upset, you can generally uncover the root cause; if you feel uncomfortable in a certain situation, you don't push those feelings down.

Being well-versed in your own emotional world is needed to prevent others from swaying you. Don't let others gaslight you into thinking you aren't feeling what you're feeling.

- You are aware of your various identities, and they all make you feel positive. You can be a mother, a teacher, a CEO, a musician, a farmer, etc. There is no cap on how many identities you can assign yourself. What's more important than their quantity is their relevance to who you really are.
- You feel in control of your life. Now, this is a tricky one because, at times, life is out of our control. Major life events come up that must be dealt with, and we can find ourselves barreling toward a situation we never wanted or envisioned. Even when that happens, it is up to us to get back on track.

Taking Back Control

Big life events could derail us temporarily, but having a clear vision with defined goals helps us stay the course. I've worked with many clients whose dreams have been derailed due to sudden life events like caring for a terminally-ill loved one. Beyond time constraints, these situations take up so much mental and emotional bandwidth it can feel impossible to take on any other commitment.

There is a story from my childhood about crossing a rushing river that has stuck with me over the years, and I believe it is an apt metaphor for when life becomes chaotic. I was ten years old and my eldest brother had taken me with him to a little island in the middle of a river near our home. We crossed the river for about 50 yards to reach a sandy beach by hopping from rock to rock. My brother's friends joined later and I decided I was ready to go home. He sent me on my way, pointing out the shallowest path across. The water moved fast and many of the rocks were slippery, but he assured me I would be okay and that he would be watching. Nonetheless, I was scared.

I carefully made my way through the water and over rocks, but about halfway back to the riverbank I lost my footing and fell into the cold water. The current washed me onto a nearby rock. I clambered out of the water and sat down, completely seized up in fear. Looking back at the island and forward to the bank, I suddenly felt alone, overwhelmed, and incapable. Here I was, in the middle of a strong current, washed away from the path to safety with no clear way back. Frankly, I was furious with my brother for putting me in this situation in the first place.

Abandoning my pride, I began to scream for help. Angry and afraid, my cries caught my brother's attention and he bolted off in my direction. I watched him leap effortlessly from rock to rock, eventually swimming up to the one I had perched myself on. He jumped out of the water and put his hand on my head, giving me a little squeeze and telling me I could calm down. We paused for a moment to allow my hysterics to subside. In typical fashion of the eldest child of a family, my brother wanted to impart a lesson as we moved through the water:

"The river is the same as life. The water level will change, and the strength of the current will fluctuate, but the water will never stop flowing. You can cry on this rock all day and you'll still be stuck in the middle of the river."

Of course, this only fueled my rage at him, but at least I was no longer alone in the situation. Someone more experienced had arrived to help me out. My brother explained the plan to help calm me down:

"You got washed off the easy path, so we need to figure out how to get across. We can't swim against the current, so let's look downstream and let the river take us to the next rock."

My heart raced as we jumped into the river. The water was icy cold and I was terrified the current would suck me away. We arrived at the next rock as promised, and sat there to warm up before taking the next plunge. The rock made me feel safe and grounded. I knew the water continued to rush past me but, in that moment, I could breathe easier.

The next time we had to swim, I felt safer and more confident. When we eventually made it to the riverbank, we hiked back up to the path I would follow to our house.

You see, when life becomes chaotic, we can't stop living it; we must find ways to exist within the chaos by carving out a space, however minuscule, to regain our footing. We may need to ask for help and take a circuitous route to arrive at the final destination, but as long as we are making steps in the right direction we've got to trust the process.

Keisha was a client of mine two years into a three-year Master's degree program. Her husband had been in a terrible accident and was rendered unable to work or care for himself, requiring Keisha to not only manage his recovery but also return to an old job to make up for the lost income. She had abandoned her dreams, money was tight and she was emotionally drained.

Among the many challenges this situation presented, Keisha's main concern with me was overcoming a crippling feeling of powerlessness and a growing pattern of negative thinking. She had risen to the occasion and wouldn't have had it any other way, but at a point she did not know where to turn for help; she was paralyzed. She found herself completely sidelining her own life out of a sense of obligation to the person she loved most.

What Keisha needed in order to change her mindset was to first validate her unpleasant feelings. Her negative thoughts did not stem from bitterness or selfishness, but from authentic disappointment and a bleak outlook on the future she had envisioned. It was okay to feel desperate and even angry. We needed to break the situation into manageable chunks to create a fresh perspective of these new circumstances. Instead of looking at the bigger picture, we looked at small ways to restore a sense of agency in her life. This resulted in her enlisting family members to help with the care of her husband, coming to an arrangement with her Master's program to complete her coursework online, and even taking time for herself to see friends again. She found small ways to feel comfort in the midst of all the pain.

We are largely in control of our own future, but we are subject to time and chance as well. Giving yourself time to mourn, grieve, and regroup is necessary, but there comes a moment when we must reestablish, and possibly modify, our original goals and vision. Even in an all-consuming situation, we must find a rock that can shield us from the chaos.

Training Assertiveness

Before we get to the part where you unleash your assertiveness, let's pinpoint one thing: there's a distinct line between assertiveness and aggression. Assertiveness has everything to do with communicating your wants and needs while respecting the wants and needs of others. Aggressiveness, on the other hand, comes from a desire to control. To be assertive is to confidently express yourself while listening to others. Aggressiveness is disrespectful and features one person placing the importance of their desires over the wants and needs of someone else. Many of us confuse asserting ourselves with being aggressive, so it is important to differentiate the two.

On the other end of that spectrum, we have passiveness, a chronic characteristic in people who tend to avoid conflict. Again, this stems from them not being confident in their individuality—as if their needs and wants are always less important than others'.

You might convey passive behavior if you say things such as "no, it's okay—you decide this time," except it isn't just that one time and you might actually say this more often. In your mind, you don't feel strongly about the choice presented to you. Or you're simply too afraid of getting a negative response. Doing this too often may cause people to start thinking that it's okay to make your decisions for you. Furthermore, it sends out the message that your needs can be freely bulldozed by someone else. Being too passive hurts you in the long run.

It may seem difficult for someone who has become accustomed to passive behavior to suddenly flip a switch. Many people have a naturally passive personality and that quality serves them well! Being decisive and able to assert yourself with confidence, however, is an essential skill set in life and in setting boundaries. Here are a few things you can do to get going:

- Voice a dissenting opinion about a non-controversial topic.

- Be simple and direct.
- Leave negative emotions out of it.
- Use 'I' statements to solidify the fact that you deserve to be respected.
- Don't be surprised if others react negatively to your newfound assertiveness and give them space to be upset without taking ownership of their feelings.
- Be mindful of your body language: stand tall, push your shoulders back, and try to maintain eye contact rather than look down or away.

Here are two examples of situations in which you could assert yourself more:

- **Practice being less lenient with your work life**. It seems as though the word 'boss' makes people feel as if they have power over how one spends their time. Although society reinforces this notion, no one's boss should push them around. If your boss or even other coworkers have gotten used to you picking up their slack or always being available, they will continue adding work to your pile. To fix this, let them know of your intentions in a way that respects the person but indicates that you will be making your own decisions from now on. For example, when your boss asks you to stay late for an extra thirty minutes, try providing a solution that caters better to your needs. For example, you could say something along the lines of "Unfortunately I can't stay in longer today. I have some personal things I must tend to, but I'll be glad to pick this up tomorrow." With a response like that, you're saying 'no' in a way that doesn't burn any bridges. You're not asking permission to do this task tomorrow, you are posing a reasonable solution that respects both your time and the work that needs to be done.
- **Stand up to your loved ones in disagreements.** Yes, sometimes it's easier to let conversations flow naturally and not even get involved with your own opinions. However, to get

comfortable with being assertive, you have to practice speaking up in *all* situations. If your family members are having a discussion about something and are presenting opinions different from yours, force yourself to chime in. No, I'm not encouraging you to instigate fights or heated arguments. Simply allow others to get accustomed to respecting your opinion. You could say, "I see what you are saying, but I actually see it differently". The key here is to keep the focus on your opinion rather than disagreeing with their point of view. Speak from your perspective by using "I" and "me". As long as you stay respectful and do not denigrate the opinions of others, you can always establish your assertiveness.

There's no reason to be ashamed of a lack of assertiveness, considering that it isn't completely natural to the majority of people. As a child, you almost always have to say 'yes'—to your parents, your teachers, or any other people superior to you. Many of us carry this passiveness well into adulthood.

The Art of Saying No without Guilt

Saying 'no' is hard. It can make you feel guilty, embarrassed, and leave you feeling like you're letting someone down. But, in reality, saying no rarely leads to battles or blood feuds. And it's more common and less risky than you think.

The art of saying no has everything to do with getting comfortable with 'no' and experiencing that saying no isn't as bad as you might have envisioned it. The more comfortable we get with it, the easier it will become, trust me.

We often feel guilty when we say 'no', because we feel responsible for the other person's reaction. We would rather avoid any conflict that might occur, safeguarding ourselves from a big fight, being made to feel selfish, or even worse, someone leaving us. In reality, however, saying 'no' to others and 'yes' to ourselves is perceived as a strength. When people are comfortable saying 'no' when needed, it elicits tremendous respect from those around them. They tend to be described as more reliable and dependable than their over-extended counterparts. Their 'yes' carries more weight as a result.

Guilt arises when we have done something wrong. Unearned guilt, however, is a concept those of us with difficulty setting boundaries are susceptible to. This is when one feels guilty about something they are not responsible for.

There are several reasons we succumb to unearned guilt, both internal and external. Some of us feel naturally responsible for the well-being of certain people in our lives, effectively blurring the line between empathy and guilt. An example of this would be allowing a friend going through a difficult time to lean on you to the point you need to cut other commitments out of your schedule. Others may experience being guilt-tripped as a result of unhealthy relationship dynamics. No matter the root source of unearned guilt, it is crucial to examine the validity of that feeling. True guilt only applies when we have violated another person's well-being due to a situation we have created. To release ourselves from the burden of guilt we must change the story we tell ourselves.

Based on what you've read so far, do you believe that forming boundaries makes you selfish? Does creating a boundary constitute some action that will result in a harmful outcome? Or is it perhaps a lack of boundaries that has you taking responsibility for a problem you did not create?

To help you on your way with saying 'no', there are a couple of things you can start doing:

- **Start noticing how often we say 'no'.** On rare occasions, someone gets angry when someone else says 'no'. If you make it a habit to start noticing how normal it is to say 'no' in conversations, you will see that it seldom leads to anger and rage. By consciously bringing your attention to these indistinct interactions, you are telling your mind that saying 'no' doesn't have to be problematic.

- **Make a counterproposal.** We don't always have to say 'no'. Sometimes it's just a matter of changing the request. When someone asks us to do something we might think we only have two options, responding with *yes* or *no*. By making a counteroffer to a request we take back control and insert our own needs. That could look something like this: "I would love to help you move this weekend, but I can only help you for two hours."
- **Buy yourself time.** If someone asks us to do something, we are not required to answer immediately. Buying time is a great way to alleviate yourself from making hasty decisions. Simply saying "I'll think about it," or "Let me get back to you on that," will immediately increase your sense of control. 'Maybe' is also an acceptable answer when you are unsure if you genuinely have the time to commit to their request.
- **Having a rule about something.** I personally use this one very often, especially when it comes to touchy topics. When someone asks you to borrow money it can be hard to answer with a blunt 'no'. Saying something like "I'm sorry I have a rule about not lending money" or "I'm sorry I can't come, we always have family dinner on Thursday nights" adds weight to your 'no'. Being told something is non-negotiable has a powerful effect. Try it out and see how disarming this simple statement can be.

Saying 'no' takes practice and it might feel uncomfortable in the beginning, but you'll see how fast it'll become your second nature once you get used to it. Get used to saying "this is non-negotiable" if you find yourself being pushed around.

Having Tough Conversations

Even if you might be the shyest person you know, the best way to handle difficult conversations is to just rip the band-aid off. In this case, it means you need to face the conversation head-on. Trust me, tiptoeing about what you truly want to say will only increase your nervousness in the moment.

Try bringing up a minor issue that bothered you by being objective and clear. Make sure you understand *why* you are bringing this issue up. Yes, your feelings may have been hurt or perhaps you felt disrespected, but what is the goal you're trying to achieve? Do you seek validation? Or are you looking for a change in the other person's behavior?

When I started out setting healthy boundaries and needed to have hard conversations, I would always prepare before I talked to the other person. It helped me calm down, gather my thoughts, center myself, and even solidify my sense of self-worth. I defined my goal for the conversation and examined my emotions, validating my reason for bringing the matter up in the first place. Once prepared, I would take a walk, go to a park, or have a cup of coffee; anything that would help me speak from a place of calm. By preparing and expelling any strong emotions before the conversation, I found myself speaking more confidently.

Let's go over how a conversation about boundaries should unfold:

1. You find a time that is comfortable for both you and the other person. Make sure the time you've scheduled to talk is adequately long and isn't immediately following a stressful day at work, for example. You want both parties to be in emotionally stable moods to perceive the conversation objectively.
2. You start by saying you have come to the conclusion that this conversation is necessary for the two of you to continue the relationship in a healthy manner. You should add that you haven't been satisfied with how things are going, and the objective of this conversation is to resolve these issues—not to attack the other person out of spite.
3. Be very clear about the boundaries you have chosen to set. In other words, don't leave them up to interpretation. Instead of using phrases sounding like "I think what could be good is...", which make your opinions sound more like passive

suggestions, say "what I need to change in order to feel good in this relationship is...".

4. Explain the reasoning behind your boundaries. In this case, the explanation is not offered as justification, but as a means for the other person to recognize why this change is required of them. Make sure not to downplay the effect of the other person's previous actions; say "when you do things like that, I feel unheard, hurt, and disrespected. I don't want to feel those things around someone I care so much about, which is why I'm introducing these boundaries and asking for a change."

5. Answer questions, as long as they are being asked respectfully. If the other person needs some further clarification on a certain boundary, provide it to them. After all, you both want to leave this conversation on the same exact page. After you've explained what your boundaries are and why you are setting them, you can discuss the details such as when they apply and how you would like them to handle these changes.

6. Listen to the other person without excusing them. When you've laid out your side, the person you're talking to might want to provide their perspective. You can listen to what they have to say and notice if they are taking accountability. If all you hear are excuses and justifications, they are likely avoiding this chance to confront their own flaws. In such a case, you will want to steer the conversation back to how their actions made you feel in the past. Make it clear you are not seeking an apology or an explanation. You simply want to maintain this relationship but need to see some changes if it is to continue.

7. If they have been responding positively and have acknowledged the past in the way you've described it, consider opening up the conversation to their boundaries as well. If it feels right, ask the person if there are any insufficient aspects of the relationship from *their* point of view and listen to them with the same understanding they offered you.

8. Make sure you both have fully understood the new requirements for the relationship and feel free to end the conversation.

The bottom line of the conversation is asserting your needs. The goal is for you to lead the conversation from a place of compassion and remain in the driver's seat. It will surely be difficult to initiate a conversation like this, and it could easily be derailed if the other person is focused on explaining or excusing their behavior - or worse, invalidating what you are attempting to tell them. Ideally, you both leave the conversation with a deeper understanding of each other as individuals and resolute to improve upon the relationship. This won't always be the case, so what can you do when your assertiveness is met with disrespect? You have, after all, found the courage to be vulnerable by expressing your feelings. It is important to realize that by allowing yourself to be vulnerable, you are also tapping into the vulnerabilities of the other person. This type of conversation could be met with defensiveness, hurt, or aggression if the other person is not ready to address some of the difficult feelings this brings up.

It is important to understand that their reaction isn't your responsibility. You initiated a conversation from a place of compassion with the intention of bettering the relationship. Any negative reaction to that could be a form of resistance, stem from their own personal issues, or simply because they're having a bad day. My point here is that there are plenty of possible reasons why they might be angry, hurt, or defensive, and those possible reasons are valid, but their reaction is not something for you to solve. If the conversation gets too heated, you can always firmly set another boundary "This is non-negotiable. I will not be yelled at, let's continue this conversation when you are ready to talk."

Key Takeaways

- To stop over-compromising it is important to make doing things for yourself a priority.
- Major life events can drag us completely off course, but there is always help and an alternative route to get you back on track.
- Setting boundaries requires confidence as well as assertiveness
- Developing assertiveness requires small changes in the way you respond to people.

- Assertiveness is exercised when you stop being lenient with others' demands, stand up for your own opinions, and learn to say 'no.'
- Having difficult conversations requires understanding and patience from both parties.
- Accept the outcome of your conversation regardless of the other person's reaction; the only goal for now is that you clearly assert yourself.

Chapter 8
Sticking to Your Boundaries

"Do not justify, apologize for, or rationalize the healthy boundary you are setting. Do not argue. Just set the boundary calmly, firmly, clearly, and respectfully."

— *Crystal Andrus*

You've found the courage to initiate a difficult conversation with someone you care about. You took an important step toward preserving the relationship by voicing your needs. Pat yourself on the back because this is something some of us will never find the strength to do! Reactions will vary and you may find yourself navigating a period of instability as this sinks in with those around you. It is possible that one conversation is all it takes with some people, yet others may challenge your assertiveness or find difficulty upholding your requests.

Old habits die hard! Your work is probably not over after that first conversation and you may have to continuously reinforce the boundary you have set. Be patient with those around you but firm in your resolve.

Time and experience will impart greater confidence if you stick to your guns.

Noticing the Changes

Most people are neither completely good nor totally bad. Helpful and destructive, vulnerable yet powerful, capable of both inflicting and feeling pain, we are complex beings unable to be labeled by a simplistic binary of good or evil. We can acknowledge that good people sometimes do bad things, and vice versa.

Our personalities are not static, and certain characteristics will be enhanced or suppressed depending on our environment. A particular work culture may develop leadership skills while suppressing creativity. A certain person may bring out your sense of humor but you have trouble being serious around them. The interplay between our personality and the traits of those around us creates the dynamic that defines how that relationship plays out.

It's safe to say that some personalities simply clash. Constant arguing or a general apathy toward one another makes it clear some people are just not a match and will probably never form a strong bond with each other. But what about a family relationship that has soured? Or a romantic relationship that started off great but has recently begun taking more from you than it gives? Perhaps a manager or colleague has become difficult to work with, yet you must find a way to carry on. It's easy to avoid becoming close with people who are clearly not a match, but when you begin asserting yourself and establishing boundaries in the later stages of a relationship, conflict may arise.

When you begin setting boundaries, telling people 'no', and asserting your opinions, you'll receive a wide array of reactions from those around you. Relationship dynamics are bound to change as your newfound confidence manifests.

Some people will become super fans and compliment you on the fact that you've found your voice. Others may react with ambivalence. And then there are those who will begin to pull away, behave (passive) aggressively toward you, or otherwise create a palpable tension in the air. Pay close attention to the changes occurring around you - who treats you differently and how?

To Be With or Not to Be With

We all know that relationships aren't always completely gratifying. Some of us might even consider leading a more solitary life because of it. After all, why expend all that emotional effort attempting to bond with a person whose presence in your life isn't necessary in the first place? Maybe it's easier to not have any friends, cut all ties with your family, and quit looking for a romantic partner.

I can't say it isn't tempting at times to simply shut everyone out. When you're feeling overwhelmed and it feels as though some of your close relationships are going through a tumultuous period, the idea of being left alone might seem heavenly. We are, however, social creatures largely incapable of a solitary existence. We need to work through our issues because the benefits of human connection far outweigh the alternative.

No one's going to be a perfect person—there will be times when they might be unintentionally cold, fail to be there for you, and even lack the willingness to have a heartfelt conversation. It would be unrealistic to expect perfection, but if any relationship causes you more stress than fulfillment, it might be time to reevaluate.

Maintaining Boundaries

Let's discuss what it takes to achieve a lasting change. You've accomplished the first step: vocally asserting your needs. What's required to maintain this new dynamic is enforcing the consequences when your boundaries continue to be overstepped.

Here are four tactics you can apply:

Restating the boundary

When someone goes back on what you agreed upon, you may need to reassert where you draw the line. You were right to speak up and you maintain the right to hold someone to their word. If you notice yourself excusing violations of your boundaries as no big deal, you are slipping back into old habits. Part of the process of maintaining your boundaries is giving them the same priority they had during the initial conversation. You won't sound like a broken record by reminding anyone to respect a boundary. You have placed the onus on them to change their behavior, so repeating your assertion out loud reinforces the issue's importance and proves your resolve. Your mindset will benefit from the double-edged effect of this as well. By asking for a small commitment from someone repeatedly, you will feel increasingly justified in your request.

Enforcing the Consequences

Eventually, enough is enough. If someone continuously oversteps a boundary even after repeated reminders, it is time to create space between you and them. It should be clear by now that this boundary is rock-solid and you will not waver. Let them know that this is the last time you will discuss this boundary with them and inform them of the consequences if they cross the line again. For example, you could say something like "If you break plans with me by not showing up or informing me, I won't go out with you anymore."

Dealing With the Bad

You have begun setting boundaries, standing up for yourself, and taking back control of your life. It may become clear at this point that some relationships will not be able to develop in the way you would have envisioned. That's okay because you have done the hard work of assessing that relationship, shown vulnerability by communicating your deepest feelings, and given someone the opportunity to work with you toward a healthier coexistence.

Let's say you have fully assessed an individual with whom you have a fraught relationship and have concluded their influence over your life must end. They continue to disregard your autonomy, it's clear you won't be able to work together to improve, and they over-exert their influence to negative effects. Clearly, they're not respecting your boundaries which is detrimental for your growth and potentially even your health. You might feel betrayed, neglected, and you just can't be yourself around this person.

Here we'll explore some tactics for dealing with a relationship that is not progressing, despite all your best efforts:

- **Take a break.** Sometimes we need a little space to evaluate whether or not a relationship is worth maintaining. Removing a person from your life for a brief period of time gives you the space to reflect on the relationship and that individual from an objective lens. Although *taking a break* is typically associated with romantic partners, you would be equally justified telling a friend or relative you need some space. It doesn't need to be a drawn-out conversation; you could simply make yourself less available. If you feel any explanation is needed, I would suggest keeping it simple - you need to focus on other things for the time being.
- **Let the relationship fade.** There could be a fine line between disengaging emotionally and becoming passive-aggressive, depending on how this is accomplished. I am not advocating the latter. Instead, remove yourself emotionally or restrict the amount of time you commit, and observe how you feel once this distance has been created. Does the extra space alleviate any stress you previously felt? What, if anything, has changed in the way you treat each other? Is there increased tension or a newfound sense of peace? The end goal is to invest your time in mutually beneficial relationships that empower you. By focusing on the healthy relationships in your life you will naturally have less time for those who do not contribute to your happiness.

- **Make a clean break.** Sometimes we hold on to people because we feel trapped by the fear of losing them. Even when we're not happy in this particular moment, we dread the loneliness we will feel without this person in our life. Yes, there will be a grieving process and you will have to pick up the pieces. You may even find yourself temporarily paralyzed by loneliness after making this decision. We crave familiarity and oftentimes it is easier to put ourselves on autopilot to endure an unhealthy situation simply because it's what we know. Realize that you are deserving of healthy love. Remind yourself that you're not alone, you still have other people around you, and that you're actively moving forward toward a better, brighter future in which you can finally be yourself. You are making space for the healthy relationships in your life to blossom, and those relationships will support you as you move through this difficult moment.

Self-Awareness

As you gain a better understanding of what you need and how to form healthier relationships, you will consequently become more aware of other people's boundaries. Awareness that we, too, can be guilty of overstepping someone else's limits can open the door to improving every relationship in our life.

Are you respecting the boundaries set by others? Acknowledging how difficult it can be to communicate a defined set of boundaries, you might consider whether others in your life could benefit from lobbing a bit of assertiveness in your direction! Admittedly a pointed question: are there any relationships in your life that might be strained by your inability to detect where a boundary exists? Don't overthink it, but you now possess the requisite knowledge to forge healthy relationships built on mutual respect, which gives you a wider perspective.

Self-awareness is developed through your sense of self and accepting the fact you are not and can never be perfect—it's normal and human if someone has a slight issue with you. If you feel that you are self-aware enough to accept your flaws, the next step is addressing them with the help of an outside perspective.

If in question, try asking those around you how happy *they* are with your relationship. Remember to have an open mind and show respect for the opinions they voice. If their experience of the relationship differs from yours, that's okay—it's exactly what this conversation is meant to uncover. Listen to their issues, try to understand their limits, and exert an effort to respect them from this point forward.

Key Takeaways

- Setting boundaries with others is no small feat, so allow yourself to be proud of the steps you've taken to improve your relationships and your life.
- Consistency is key, make sure the person upholds their end of the deal and respects your boundaries continuously.
- Reinforce your boundaries with actions - impose consequences if a boundary is repeatedly violated.
- If someone chooses to not comply with your boundaries, it might be time to end the relationship. Take the time to grieve while acknowledging the fact that it needed to end. Stick to your non-negotiables.
- Apply your knowledge of boundaries to see if there are people in your life who may want to set some boundaries with you as well.

Chapter 9
Enjoying a Fresh Take on Life

You never change your life until you step out of your comfort zone; change begins at the end of your comfort zone.

— *Roy T. Bennett*

It's not easy, but once you take the steps prescribed in this book to set clear boundaries, prepare to reap the rewards! You'll feel a newfound sense of freedom. You'll have time to start up that hobby, side hustle, or passion project that's been sitting on the shelf collecting dust, and the people surrounding you push you forward and support you on this journey. There are certain to be bumps along the way, but your new mindset on how to approach them sees the promise of mental peace at the end of the bumpy road. By seeing our obstacles as opportunities, we turn our problems into progress.

Growth in Discomfort

I'm willing to bet a number of the tactics discussed throughout this book strike you as extremely uncomfortable propositions. It is not easy to depart from the well-trodden path in favor of blazing our own trail toward personal growth. Confronting the inner demons that enable the people around us to overstep our boundaries is not a pleasant task. But growth does not come from a place of comfort. Comfort and growth do not coexist. The way I see it, we're only given two options: spend a lackluster existence living up to the expectations of others, or embrace the challenges and face life head-on.

There's a saying "If you keep doing what you're doing, you'll keep getting what you're getting". Our actions perpetuate themselves, so if we allow someone to violate a boundary once, they are destined to continue doing so. Take the power into your hands by showing you have clear limits about what you'll tolerate, and watch everything else fall into line. Dare to dream big, dare to disagree, and take ownership of your journey. The goal in your path toward personal growth is not to eradicate discomfort, it is to get comfortable with being uncomfortable.

Change often induces fear. Fear of being pulled out of our comfort zone, leaving us fully exposed and vulnerable. However, if we take the metaphor of a hermit crab, we get a better understanding of how discomfort can be a catalyst for growth. Hermit crabs are curious little creatures that shed their exoskeleton several times throughout their lives in a process called *molting*. During this process, the crab's body has grown too big, making it uncomfortable to stay in its shell. They are easy prey and incredibly vulnerable as they seek a new home that fits their larger body. Like the example of the hermit crab, we must allow ourselves to get uncomfortable and put ourselves in danger by 'coming out of our shells', but it is only through this process that we achieve actual growth.

An Oath to Truth

We discussed the two basic human needs of connection and authenticity at the beginning of this book. When those two needs are in balance, we are happy in our lives and in our relationships. We feel the freedom to be ourselves without compromising deep connections with others. People who enjoy the balance of authenticity and connectedness display confidence, good habits, and healthy relationships - all of which fuel the fire to continue improving upon what's already working.

Authenticity is not an endpoint. Rather, it is an ongoing process of being truthful to ourselves in every single moment. It takes constant attention to the root of what makes you, *you* - and focusing on that truth as your north star. Authenticity is not something we need to create or discover. Though we may have buried it deep within, it is merely the truth that exists at the core of our being.

We often praise and value the honesty of children. We attribute it to their innocence and purity and might even say "I wish I could be more like that". Once as a little girl, I looked across the table at Thanksgiving dinner and proclaimed "Aunt Mary got fat!" to the shock and horror of my parents. They immediately and harshly corrected my behavior as everyone turned to observe how Aunt Mary would react. She chuckled with great warmth, looked at me, and said "It's true! I have gotten fatter since I last visited". She wasn't offended because we expect children to speak outrageous truths as they are learning to observe the world around them.

Somewhere down the line, however, we lose that. We are taught it's better to tell a white lie to spare someone's feelings. The more we experience positive feedback as a result of our white lies, the better we get at telling them. Likewise, the more we observe the negative feedback when voicing the truth, the better we get at suppressing it.

Now I'm not romanticizing a childlike innocence or proposing that kind of response to our surroundings as adults. We have the mental capacity to choose our words more carefully and avoid unnecessary conflict and hurt feelings. But instead of lying to someone to keep the peace, we can opt for truthful alternatives.

A dear friend of mine is an actress and recently invited me to her latest play. I find her to be a talented actress and it brings me great joy to support my friend's artistic endeavor while she struts her stuff on stage. Aside from the chance to see her perform, however, the play was perhaps one of the worst I've ever had to sit through. I lit up every time she came out on the stage and she delivered a great performance, in my (honest) opinion. The play itself, however, was a dud (in my humble opinion).

We went out for drinks after the show and I was momentarily at a loss for the right words. When my friend eventually asked, "And, what did you think?" I could have been honest and told her the show failed to keep my attention, the set design was ugly and the lead actor couldn't hold a note. But it wouldn't have fit the moment and I'm no theater critic anyway. She was clearly thrilled to be part of this show and landing this role was a big accomplishment for her.

My dilemma was how to live up to my oath of truth while not hurting her feelings or belittling her achievement. So I dug deep - I had not gone to the show because I had high expectations of a life-changing theatrical experience; I had gone to see my friend do what she does best, and she nailed it. So I decided on this truth: "I loved seeing you perform, you nailed this role and I am so thrilled you asked me to come."

I didn't feel I was betraying my authenticity by simply focusing on the positive in order to connect with my friend over an achievement she was proud of. Her need for validation is what that moment called for, so we celebrated her success. There came a later conversation where we discussed the merits of the play itself and I was happily honest because she had invited me to share my opinion.

Discovering Yourself

The gift I hope you receive from reading this book is the gift of a greater self-understanding and a sense of integrity toward your true self. When we embrace our authenticity we create a current that allows life to flow in the direction it was always meant to go.

Learning to set boundaries allows your authenticity the space to breathe freely. It is about taking off the mask and becoming confident in your vulnerability. You will become more daring to try new things and might even transform into an entirely different version of *you* - a version you had only dreamt of before. When we hide behind a mask, people can only comment on that mask, so we cannot possibly feel *seen* or fully understood.

By daring to share what truly lights your fire, you allow others the opportunity to profoundly connect with the *real* you. Some will add fuel to the fire and support your growth. Others may try to extinguish it and keep you but a glowing ember full of potential. It is through self-discovery that we can more easily identify the people who fuel our fire and become innately aware of the boundaries needed to protect it.

With integrity to your true self, you become comfortable with being uncomfortable. You stop allowing fear to cloud your judgment of what you know to be right and wrong. You know who you are and what you need.

Listening to Your Intuition

Getting more in tune with your true self will awaken your inner voice. It is that little voice that has been trying to tell you what's right all along. In the process of self-discovery, you will notice your intuition speaking louder and more often as it guides you toward choices, people, and situations that are likely to have a positive impact.

Not to be confused with instinct, which is a one-dimensional pattern of behavior that influences your decision-making, intuition sprouts from the authentic self. Instinct is a natural, hardwired tendency to behave or react in a certain way. Intuition is a deeper understanding. It is the expression of our emotional, spiritual and logical sides all working in perfect harmony.

Intuition is our built-in GPS that is in touch with our true desires and needs and maps out the best path toward them. It tells us: *'just quit that job you hate already!'*, or *'start writing that book you've been fantasizing about'*. But our logical mind takes over in an effort to protect us. We tend to succumb to the fear of failure. We doubt ourselves and become judgemental of our 'crazy' ideas.

Only by actively listening to our intuition do we come closer to a sense of happiness and fulfillment. Ask yourself this: What makes my heart jump? How does it feel once I've embraced that and succeeded? What new doors are opened because of this leap of faith? Do I dare to be bold enough to embrace this dream and make it a reality?

Your brain will present you with fear, shame, and judgment in a valiant yet misguided attempt at self-preservation. Instead, I suggest putting your logical side to work and come up with a set of practical goals that lead you, step by step, toward the dream life you desire.

Key Takeaways

- Healthy and valuable relationships allow you to flourish and grow as a person.
- Improving your life often means getting comfortable with discomfort; step out of your comfort zone to unlock new possibilities.
- Consistent honesty brings us closer to our authentic selves.
- Learning to set boundaries allows your authenticity to thrive.
- Through intuition we already know what we truly desire and need. We just have to be brave enough to listen to it.

Conclusion

Trust yourself, you have survived a lot, and you will survive whatever is coming.

— Robert Tew

I want you to trust yourself. Yes, I can share with you the lessons my own life has taught me, things I've seen other people learn, and the facts that I have come to rely on throughout my professional career, but nothing beats your own intuition, guided by a true understanding of your authentic self. Much of what was written in the past nine chapters is likely something you already know deep down. Sometimes, we might just need someone else to deliver the message in order for it to fully sink in.

The fear that arises when we think about change in our lives often has nothing to do with external factors. Much of the fear we feel about our future has nothing to do with scary possibilities outside of our control. It has everything to do with being afraid of a version of ourselves we don't yet know. We are comfortable when we know who we are; when considering big changes we give up that comfort. We have to agree to abandon this version of ourselves for a new one, which can be terrifying.

A sense of responsibility to be kind and selfless should enrich your life, not make it miserable. If we have grown comfortable allowing people to mistreat us time and again, it will be difficult to confront the reasons why we have tolerated their undue influence over our lives. By firmly asserting our boundaries, we clear up space in our hearts and our minds for the seeds of positivity to sprout. You can be so caught up in pleasing the people who will never truly value your efforts that you might actually miss the people you have been hoping to meet all your life. Do not put yourself in such a position—make that space for yourself.

Realize the power you have to change any situation. It doesn't matter if you don't feel ready, because remember: discomfort is your superpower. The more you accept it and fit it into your life in a healthy way, the easier it will be to handle. Free yourself from the fear of becoming a more powerful *you*. Start living your life through conscious action, even if it means giving up the reality you are used to.

Bibliography

20 inspirational quotes on boundaries. Jane Taylor | Mindfulness & Compassion Teacher | Mind-Body Connection Coach | Wellbeing Coaching | Mindful Self-Compassion Coaching | Gold Coast. (2021, October 18). https://www.habitsforwellbeing.com/20-inspirational-quotes-on-boundaries/

Ackerman, C. E. (2018, November 6). *What is self-worth & how do we build it? (incl.. worksheets).* PositivePsychology.com. Retrieved September 22, 2022, from https://positivepsychology.com/self-worth/#what-is

Borreli, L. (2016, March 2). *People-pleaser: Brain scans show pushovers agree with others to avoid mental stress.* Medical Daily. Retrieved September 22, 2022, from https://www.medicaldaily.com/people-pleaser-brain-activity-mental-stress-376139

Brandt, A. (2018, April 2). *9 steps to healing childhood trauma as an adult.* Psychology Today. Retrieved September 22, 2022, from https://www.psychologytoday.com/ca/blog/mindful-anger/201804/9-steps-healing-childhood-trauma-adult

Cherry, K. (2021, September 3). *How to stop being a people-pleaser.* Verywell Mind. Retrieved September 22, 2022, from https://www.verywellmind.com/how-to-stop-being-a-people-pleaser-5184412

Conley, M. (2022, March 28). *45 quotes that celebrate teamwork, hard work, and collaboration.* HubSpot Blog. Retrieved September 22, 2022, from https://blog.hubspot.com/marketing/teamwork-quotes

Firestone, T. (2018, May 4). *Preserving individuality to strengthen your relationship.* PsychAlive. Retrieved September 22, 2022, from https://www.psychalive.org/preserving-individuality-strengthen-relationship/

Goodreads. (n.d.). *A quote by Dido Stargaze.* Goodreads. Retrieved October 4, 2022, from https://www.goodreads.com/quotes/10881157-if-your-absence-doesn-t-bother-them-then-your-presence-never

Goodreads. (n.d.). *A quote by Shannon L. Alder.* Goodreads. Retrieved October 4, 2022, from https://www.goodreads.com/quotes/706138-the-only-real-conflict-you-will-ever-have-in-your

Goodreads. (n.d.). *Boundaries Quotes (451 quotes).* Goodreads. Retrieved October 4, 2022, from https://www.goodreads.com/quotes/tag/boundaries#:~:text=%E2%80%9CWhen%20we%20fail%20to%20set,a%20behavior%20or%20a%20choice.%E2%80%9D

Goodreads. (n.d.). *Comfort zone quotes (342 quotes).* Goodreads. Retrieved October 4, 2022, from https://www.goodreads.com/quotes/tag/comfort-zone

Goodreads. (n.d.). *Self worth quotes (1650 quotes).* Goodreads. Retrieved October 4, 2022, from https://www.goodreads.com/quotes/tag/self-worth

Klein, Y. (2021, January 20). *How to get over a friendship breakup.* Evolve Treatment Centers. Retrieved September 22, 2022, from https://evolvetreatment.com/blog/friendship-breakup/

Lechnyr, D. (2022, June 29). *The consequences of not having any boundaries*. TherapyDave. Retrieved September 22, 2022, from https://therapydave.com/self-help/the-consequences-of-not-having-any-boundaries/

Martin, S. (2020, April 23). *7 types of boundaries you may need*. Psych Central. Retrieved September 22, 2022, from https://psychcentral.com/blog/imperfect/2020/04/7-types-of-boundaries-you-may-need

Morin, A. (2016, June 20). *Compliments make you cringe? science explains the reasons why*. Inc.com. Retrieved September 22, 2022, from https://www.inc.com/amy-morin/compliments-make-you-cringe-science-explains-the-reasons-why.html

Morin, A. (n.d.). *10 signs you're a people-pleaser*. Psychology Today. Retrieved September 22, 2022, from https://www.psychologytoday.com/ca/blog/what-mentally-strong-people-dont-do/201708/10-signs-youre-people-pleaser

Newhouse, L. (2021, March 1). *Is crying good for you?* Harvard Health. Retrieved September 22, 2022, from https://www.health.harvard.edu/blog/is-crying-good-for-you-2021030122020#:~:text=Researchers%20have%20established%20that%20crying,both%20physical%20and%20emotional%20pain.

Nitka, D. (2020, August 7). *The importance of setting boundaries*. Connecte Psychology. Retrieved September 22, 2022, from https://connectepsychology.com/en/2017/05/16/the-importance-of-setting-boundaries/#:~:text=In%20the%20context%20of%20psychology,adult%20is%20responsible%20for%20themselves.

Prism Health North Texas. (n.d.). Establishing healthy boundaries. Retrieved from http://www.prismhealthntx.org/establishing-healthy-boundaries/

Pangilinan, J. (2022, February 24). *51 quotes about Healing your body & mind [2022 update]*. Happier Human. Retrieved October 4, 2022, from https://www.happierhuman.com/quotes-about-healing/

Quotations, S. Q. (n.d.). *The greatest value of having good people around you is not what you get from them but the better person you become because of them... - searchquotes*. Search Quotes. Retrieved October 4, 2022, from https://www.searchquotes.com/quotation/The_greatest_value_of_having_good_people_around_you_is_not_what_you_get_from_them_but_the_better_per/509245/

Santos-Longhurst, A. (2022, March 31). *How to identify your love language*. Healthline. Retrieved September 22, 2022, from https://www.healthline.com/health/love-languages

Subjects. CliffsNotes. (n.d.). Retrieved September 22, 2022, from https://www.cliffsnotes.com/cliffsnotes/subjects/literature/in-which-play-did-william-shakespeare-state-that-misery-loves-company#:~:text=From%2019th%2Dcentury%20American%20essayist,%2C%20misery%20has%20company%20enough.%22

Team, T. S. (2022, September 21). *50 life-changing quotes about trusting yourself*. The STRIVE. Retrieved October 4, 2022, from https://thestrive.co/quotes-about-trusting-yourself/

Waytz, A. (n.d.). *Friend or foe? A psychological perspective on trust*. Friend or Foe? The Psychology of Trust | The Trust Project. Retrieved September 22, 2022, from https://www.kellogg.northwestern.edu/trust-project/videos/waytz-ep-1.aspx

Willis, J., & Todorov, A. (2006, July). *First Impressions: Making up your mind after a 100-MS ... - sage journals*. Retrieved September 23, 2022, from https://journals.sagepub.com/doi/10.1111/j.1467-9280.2006.01750.x

Xplore. (n.d.). *Barbara de Angelis quotes*. BrainyQuote. Retrieved October 4, 2022, from https://www.brainyquote.com/quotes/barbara_de_angelis_119456?src=t_relationship
Xplore. (n.d.). *Marcus Tullius Cicero quotes*. BrainyQuote. Retrieved October 4, 2022, from https://www.brainyquote.com/quotes/marcus_tullius_cicero_156298#

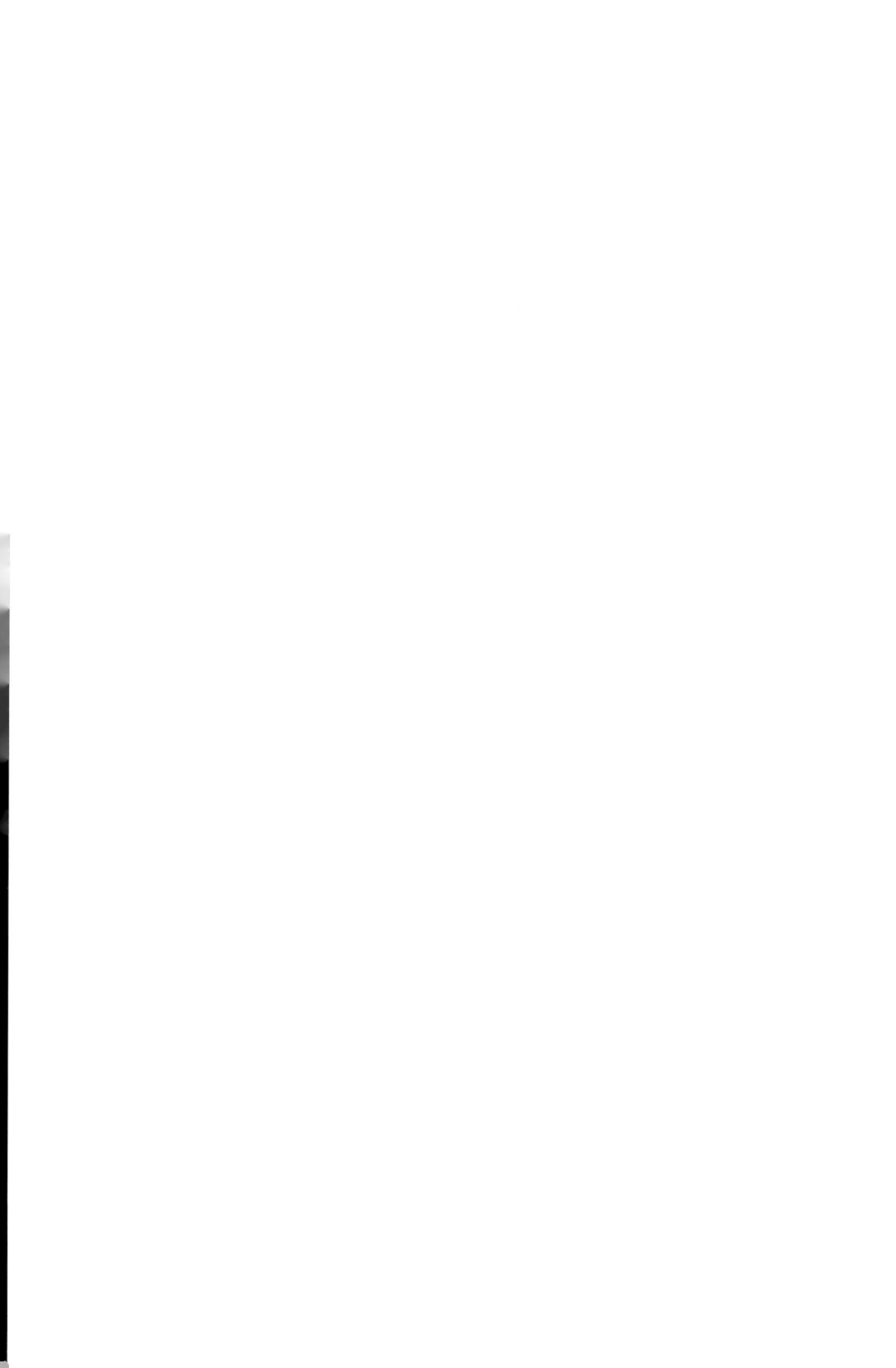

The Proven Path to Self-Compassion

Discover the Power of Self-Love, Self-Care and Mindfulness

Introduction

Throughout our lives, we learn to show sympathy and support our loved ones when they're feeling unworthy or facing challenging times. We know how to ask "What do you need?", offer help, and reassure them that they always can count on us. We speak gently and with kindness, using nonverbal cues like a warm embrace or a steady hand on their shoulder to show we care. And when necessary, we take swift and decisive action to protect our loved ones. We feel a surge of energy when they are in danger and need our protection, and we help them overcome obstacles with a little nudge. Through experience, we have mastered the insight and skills to be there for others in all kinds of situations.

Unfortunately, we don't often show ourselves the same compassion and understanding when faced with adversity. Instead of pausing to ask ourselves what we need in the moment and providing comfort and support, we may be more prone to judgment, problem-solving, or panic. When we spill coffee on our way to work, we instantly berate ourselves for being too clumsy or stupid. But would we ever do that to a close friend? It's interesting to note how frequently we speak to ourselves in this negative way and yet still find ways to justify it.

Self-criticism and unattainable standards prevent us from giving ourselves the respect we deserve, stifling our emotions and leaving us feeling unsafe and lonely. When we are hard on ourselves, we go into defense mode. We can't make a mistake, or else we'll shower ourselves with insults. What some of us are not realizing is that this constant stream of low-level stress is harming our minds, hearts, and bodies.

Believing that survival depends on maintaining perfect control over every aspect of our lives might trap us in an endless circle of suffering. It has the potential to paralyze us, preventing us from going after our goals. Overwhelmed by negative thoughts and feelings, we may act in ways inconsistent with our ideals, leading to more self-criticism and perpetuating the cycle of negativity. By failing to acknowledge the damage we cause by our negative self-talk and succumbing to it, we risk getting stuck in a never-ending loop and ultimately losing all our self-esteem.

This type of negativity prevents us from reaching our full potential and greatly impacts our mental and emotional well-being. But we don't have to keep being our worst enemy; we can learn to be as kind to ourselves as we are to others. Imagine how much better we would feel if we could let go of those negative thoughts and treat ourselves with the same compassion.

This book offers insight into the importance of self-compassion and provides research-backed methods for developing it. By reading this book and implementing its guidance, you can work toward a more compassionate relationship with yourself. You'll learn how to manage self-criticism and cultivate self-compassion, which will decrease your levels of stress and anxiety significantly.

Self-compassion is the practice of being kind and understanding toward yourself despite your flaws and even when you make mistakes. It means recognizing that you deserve love and compassion no matter what, just like anyone else. It's a supportive inner voice that encourages you to be kind to yourself and take care of yourself. Self-compassion helps you find hope in difficult times and fully enjoy your successes in times of bliss.

Contrary to popular belief, self-compassion is not a complex mental exercise that can only be attained by monks who practiced years of meditation. It's something that we can all cultivate and train. By being kind and understanding friends to ourselves, we can develop self-compassion and experience its many benefits.

Being compassionate and caring are human tendencies that come naturally and give us a lot in return. It's not about being perfect but rather about finding ways to support ourselves and cope with life's challenges. By prioritizing self-care and happiness over perfectionism and anxiety, we develop a healthier, more compassionate, and more understanding relationship with ourselves. And while self-compassion won't solve all of our problems, it can help us to better navigate difficult times and emotions.

By showing yourself kindness and understanding, you can approach your mistakes with curiosity and with a desire to learn and improve rather than judge and blame. This can be extremely useful when you have done something you feel bad about or something that is out of alignment with your values. Instead of judging yourself harshly, you can say to yourself, "I made a mistake, but that doesn't make me a bad person, and it's just a reminder that I need to make some changes."

Take note that self-compassion is not about absolving yourself from responsibility; it's about recognizing that you are worthy of care and support even when you make mistakes and that you can make positive changes in your life at any given moment.

There may be countless new opportunities uncovered by using this strategy. Imagine how you'd feel if you went about your day knowing you deserve kindness and compassion at all times, enabling you to tackle each difficulty more positively. Think of all the possibilities that would arise in your personal and professional life if you would fully embrace this way of thinking. Our critical voice discourages us from putting ourselves out there, taking chances, and making meaningful connections with others, but self-compassion can give us the courage and confidence we so desperately need in these situations.

This book will teach you how to cultivate compassion through mindfulness techniques and other 'staying present'-strategies. By learning to let go of distractions and identifying the sources of negativity in your life, you can become kinder to yourself when it matters most. These techniques can help you become more self-aware and make you better able to respond to your own needs with compassion and care.

To get the most out of this book, approach it with the following mindset: instead of thinking of yourself as broken and in need of fixing, try viewing yourself as perfectly imperfect, just as you are. Adopting this mindset will make your experience a lot easier and more enjoyable. This book will assist you in dealing with emotional pain from a place of kindness and love.

To get good at something, you need to practice it a lot. Doing the exercises regularly and putting in the time and effort to practice self-compassion is essential. The more you practice and the more consistent you are, the better you will get at it. It's recommended to practice for at least 30 minutes daily, but if that's not possible, don't stress about it, do what feels reasonable and manageable for you.

Remember that everyone is different and what works for one person may not work for another. If something you read in this book doesn't feel helpful or valuable to you, feel free to adjust, personalize, or even skip it; a different chapter or approach may resonate with you more. I do encourage you to try everything at least once and with full dedication. What may feel cumbersome or challenging initially may eventually become liberating and helpful. Be open to trying new things and applying what you learn; you may discover valuable new ways of doing things you never deemed possible. It's also important to recognize that some exercises may bring up difficult emotions or thoughts, as they ask us to confront our challenges directly. This is a normal part of the process, but it's crucial to take care of yourself and move at a comfortable pace.

By working with this guide, you have already taken an important step toward a happier, healthier, and more self-compassionate life. Self-compassion can profoundly impact your well-being, as I have seen first-hand in my work with clients and personal experience. Through my years of practice, I have witnessed its transformative power in helping people learn to love themselves, no matter their achievements or how challenging things may be.

I am excited to support you on your journey and hope you will experience the same sense of freedom and fulfillment that my clients have found through this practice. As we embark on this journey together, I wish you the best as you actively cultivate love, warmth, kindness, compassion, and joy for yourself and others. Let's get started!

Chapter 1
What is Self-Compassion?

"Self-compassion–being supportive and kind to yourself, especially in the face of stress and failure–is associated with more motivation and better self-control."

- Kelly McGonigal

According to Buddhist teachings, self-compassion is essential to the path toward enlightenment and is seen as a way to alleviate suffering and promote happiness. When we are compassionate toward ourselves, we can accept ourselves as we are rather than constantly trying to improve or change ourselves. When we accept things as they are, we can find satisfaction and serenity in the present moment instead of becoming entangled in a cycle of pain and sorrow.

Self-compassion refers to the act of being kind and understanding toward oneself during difficult times, rather than being overly critical or judgmental. It involves treating ourselves with the same compassion and understanding that we would offer to a friend or loved one. Additionally, self-compassion is seen as a way to develop wisdom and understanding. We can see things more clearly and recognize the interconnectedness of all things and beings; this understanding leads to a greater sense of compassion for the world around us.

Empathy and Compassion

Empathy and self-compassion are the foundations of emotional intelligence, and when we can master them, we can genuinely thrive both personally and professionally. Empathy is the ability to understand and share the feelings of another person. It involves being able to perceive and respond to the emotional states of others accurately, or being able "to put ourselves in another's shoes."

Compassion involves not only understanding another person's feelings but also feeling motivated to help them somehow. It consists of the desire to alleviate suffering and offer comfort and support.

Empathy and compassion allow us to connect with others, understand their feelings, and accept our own emotions. When we can empathize with others, we build stronger relationships and create a more compassionate society.

It is possible to have empathy without feeling compassion, and vice versa. Someone empathetic may be able to understand and appreciate another person's feelings, but may not feel motivated to help them in any way. On the other hand, compassionate people may strongly desire to help others, even if they do not fully understand or share their feelings.

Turning compassion toward yourself involves taking a (pro)active approach to addressing and improving your own struggles. When we can practice self-compassion, we build inner strength and resilience, allowing us to navigate life's challenges with grace and understanding.

The Myths of Self-Compassion

Unfortunately, some common misconceptions about self-compassion discourage people from learning more about it. These misconceptions range from thinking self-compassion is the same as self-pity or laziness to believing it's not as important as self-esteem. We can take the first step toward developing self-compassion by recognizing and refuting these myths and misconceptions.

Myth: Self-compassion is selfish.

Fact: Self-compassion is the opposite of selfishness, and it involves acknowledging and accepting our own suffering, as well as the suffering of others. By being kind and understanding toward ourselves, we can be more present and available to support others.

Myth: Self-compassion is a sign of weakness.

Fact: Self-compassion is actually a sign of strength. It requires much courage to be honest with ourselves about our flaws and weaknesses.

Myth: Self-compassion is the same as self-indulgence.

Fact: Self-compassion is about finding balance. It involves taking care of ourselves and meeting our own needs; it does not mean indulging in unhealthy behaviors or neglecting our responsibilities.

Myth: Self-compassion is the same as self-pity.

Fact: Self-compassion involves acknowledging and accepting our own suffering, while self-pity involves dwelling on our suffering and feeling sorry for ourselves.

Myth: Self-compassion is easy.

Fact: Practicing self-compassion can be difficult, especially if we are used to being hard on ourselves. It requires acknowledging and accepting our flaws and weaknesses, which can be very challenging.

Myth: Self-compassion is the same as self-esteem.

Fact: While self-compassion and self-esteem are related, they are very different. Self-compassion is about treating oneself with kindness and understanding, even in difficult situations, while self-esteem is about valuing and approving ourselves. It says more about how much we think we are worth and how much we like ourselves.

Myth: Self-compassion is only for people with low self-esteem.

Fact: Self-compassion can be beneficial for people with all levels of self-esteem. It can help people with low self-esteem to feel more worthy and accepted, and it can help people with high self-esteem to be more realistic and balanced in their self-evaluations.

Myth: Self-compassion is only for people who are struggling.

Fact: While self-compassion can be especially helpful for people struggling with difficult emotions or challenges, it is not only for those struggling. Everyone can benefit from self-compassion, as it can help us feel more grounded, connected, and satisfied with our lives.

Now let's dive a little deeper into some of these misconceptions.

The Pursuit of High Self-Esteem

It's been drilled into our heads that having high self-esteem is crucial to happiness and success. But is it really that simple? Recent studies show that this constant need to view ourselves positively is backfiring on us.

Promoting high self-esteem has been trending and immensely popular for many years, with countless media outlets advocating it. However, studies reveal that pursuing high self-esteem can actually lead to an inflated sense of self-importance and a lack of empathy for others.

In a society where being average is seen as a failure, many people try to make themselves appear better than others, leading to increased levels of narcissism. In the past 20 years, this has become a serious issue, with 65%

of college students displaying higher levels of narcissism than previous generations. This constant need to feel superior can lead to feelings of loneliness and disconnection.

One of the most common misconceptions about self-compassion is that it is the same as self-esteem. Although the two concepts are sometimes intertwined, they are very different. Self-compassion is a form of self-acceptance that does not depend on a person's performance or achievements and shifts the focus from trying to be perfect to simply being content with yourself.

Self-esteem is often based on external validation and comparison to others rather than an internal sense of self-worth. When our self-worth becomes too tied to meeting other people's expectations or standards, it can lead to a constant need for validation and a fear of failure. Additionally, high self-esteem doesn't always translate to positive self-regard and doesn't protect against negative emotions, such as shame and self-doubt. It may also cause or exacerbate feelings of isolation, whereas self-compassion helps individuals to see themselves more positively and as part of a collective, resulting in a stronger sense of belonging.

It's time to shift our focus from self-esteem to self-compassion. Instead of constantly criticizing ourselves for not being enough, we can fully embrace and accept ourselves for who we are in this very moment. Let's strive for a world where you wake up every morning and look in the mirror with nothing but love and appreciation for the person staring back at you. No more negative self-talk or harsh criticisms. Just pure, unconditional acceptance.

Shaking False Beliefs

Self-pity and self-indulgence often keep us from achieving our goals and living our best lives. We feel sorry for ourselves because of our perceived failures or setbacks and fear we might become lazy when we're 'too soft' on ourselves. However, it's important to note that self-pity and self-indulgence are very different from being self-compassionate.

The entanglement of self-pity

Self-pity is a trap that can easily ensnare individuals, causing them to become consumed with their struggles and problems, unable to see that others are also struggling and experiencing difficulties. It's a state of mind that leads us to feelings of isolation and disconnection from others. People who fall into this trap often exaggerate their sorrow and become fixated on their own pain, unable to empathize with others.

On the other hand, self-kindness offers a powerful antidote to these negative emotions by helping individuals recognize the shared humanity in their pain. It enables them to see their own experiences in the context of the larger human experience and to understand that they are not alone in their pain. It can help them avoid the tendency to be overly dramatic and melodramatic about their bad luck and misfortunes.

Self-pity can make it hard to gain distance from your predicament and see things more clearly. It facilitates getting trapped in a bubble, which makes it difficult to see the bigger picture. Practicing self-compassion, however, allows you to step back and view yourself with the same empathy and understanding as an objective third party. This perspective allows you to gain a broader understanding of your situation and helps you find a way to move forward.

The Fine Line of Self-indulgence

Many of us find it challenging to be compassionate toward ourselves because we fear that we might let ourselves off the hook too much. We think being kind to ourselves is the same as indulging in unhealthy habits, like eating junk food, sleeping late, and watching too much TV. But that's not proper self-care; that's self-indulgence.

Taking care of ourselves and achieving lasting enjoyment usually entails a certain level of discomfort. Maintaining good health, developing new skills, and pursuing meaningful experiences often involves pushing ourselves out of our comfort zones, which forces us to face challenges and obstacles. Confronting these difficulties and overcoming them will allow us to grow and find a deeper sense of fulfillment and satisfaction.

Real self-compassion is about striving for long-term wellness. Giving in to instant pleasure can often be detrimental to our overall health, but genuine self-compassion is about making choices that will lead to sustainable vitality and happiness.

Chapter Takeaways

- Self-compassion is a concept borrowed from Buddhism aimed at alleviating suffering.
- Treating oneself the same kindness we would have for a best friend is at the heart of self-compassion.
- Empathy and compassion allow us to connect with others and ourselves deeply.
- There are a lot of myths and misconceptions about self-compassion that prevent us from fully reaping its benefits.
- To truly understand the concept of self-compassion, we must learn its difference from self-esteem, self-pity, and self-indulgence.

Chapter 2
The Benefits of Self-Compassion

"Practice self-compassion. Talk to and be your best, kind, compassionate, caring friend."

— *Kristin Neff*

Self-compassion is one of the most potent sources of resilience. It has many positive effects, such as lowering levels of loneliness, improving concentration, and lessening the tendency to "project" your feelings onto others. It is the antidote to self-attacking and has proven to conquer "the inner critic." It helps us tone down our self-flagellating attitudes, behaviors, and feelings that steal away our confidence and peace of mind and set off our unhealthy coping mechanisms.

By learning to be kind to ourselves, we can turn off our brain's threat system and instead turn toward our "safety/soothing system," allowing us to face our feelings head-on and react more efficiently to the trials of daily life.

Advantages of Self-Compassion

Self-compassion is a strong predictor of happiness; people who master it tend to be less depressed, less nervous, and less prone to experiencing excessive shame (or even suicide ideation). Practicing it drastically improves emotional well-being, builds a stronger sense of self-worth, develops resilience, and improves our relationships and physical health.

Let's get straight to it and have a deeper look at the many benefits of self-compassion:

Improving emotional well-being: Self-compassion has been shown to reduce symptoms of depression, anxiety, and stress. Instead of criticizing yourself or dwelling on negative thoughts, you'll learn to understand and accept your flaws and limitations, allowing you to better cope with difficult emotions like shame and guilt.

Cultivating self-kindness allows us to accept our humanity and to be more understanding and accepting of ourselves, warts and all. Instead of weakening ourselves with self-criticism and doubt, we can build ourselves up with self-compassion.

Think of it like going on an adventurous journey. You set out with high hopes and big dreams but encounter obstacles and setbacks along the way. Instead of giving up, self-compassion helps you to see these challenges as opportunities for growth and development. It's like having a trusty companion by your side, encouraging you to keep going and to take care of yourself along the way.

Enhancing self-worth: Self-compassion helps individuals to develop a more stable and healthy sense of self-worth. Unlike self-esteem, which is based on external validation, self-compassion is an unconditional form of self-acceptance. It allows you to fully accept yourself as you are, which leads to a more stable and robust sense of self-worth.

Self-worth that is solely based on having high self-esteem is predicated on competition with others and excelling at something to feel good about yourself. It is based on success and makes it easy to give up on yourself when you fail. Basing your self-worth on self-compassion means treating yourself with kindness, understanding, and acceptance, rather than constantly seeking external validation. It involves recognizing and accepting your own flaws, failures, and imperfections, while also acknowledging and embracing your strengths, accomplishments, and successes. By approaching yourself with self-compassion, you can develop a healthier, more fulfilling sense of self-worth and emotional well-being.

Facilitating personal growth: Self-compassion allows you to acknowledge your flaws and mistakes without feeling guilty or ashamed. People who are very hard on themselves may find it hard to take risks because they fear disappointment or failure. When you have less of a fear of failure, you are more willing to venture out into the unknown. You create a safe space for yourself to learn from mishaps and examine yourself lovingly, leading to healthy personal growth.

Self-compassion fosters personal growth by encouraging introspection and improving self-awareness. By attentively observing your emotions and thoughts, you gain a deeper insight into your priorities, needs, and values. This leads to a better understanding of yourself and helps you see the steps you need to take to reach your goals.

Improving relationships: Self-compassion will also have a positive impact on your relationships. It will help you to be more empathetic and understanding, and less critical and judgmental, toward others.

When it comes to relationships, it's important to remember that we can only be as kind and patient to others as we are to ourselves. That's where self-compassion comes in. Practicing self-empathy can help us to become better partners, friends, family members, colleagues, bosses, and parents. It's like a secret recipe for success in our relationships.

Imagine being more at ease with yourself, like slipping into your favorite pair of jeans. It's that comfortable, confident feeling that makes it easier to connect with others. By learning to be more self-compassionate, you'll become less self-centered and develop your capacity for empathy.

Promoting resilience: Self-compassion helps you to see your problems and difficulties from a broader perspective, which can help you to feel less overwhelmed and more resilient in the face of adversity. When you learn to be more self-compassionate, you are more likely to view challenges as opportunities for growth and development rather than overwhelming obstacles.

When failures don't seem so catastrophic and self-criticism fades into the background, you'll have more time to find pleasure in life. Mistakes and failures can be seen as learning opportunities rather than reflections of our character, which can lead to a healthier self-image and more positive outlook on life. Spending less time ruminating on past failures and failings leaves more time for the things and people you truly value.

Improving physical health: Self-compassion has been linked to a reduction in anxiety and stress on a physiological level. Self-criticism and self-judgment can trigger a "threat state," where the limbic system is heightened, and your "fight or flight" response is initiated. Constant exposure to this state has been linked to anxiety and depression.

Perhaps you have experienced the calming effect of a friend's encouraging words or comforting touch in times of hardship. We share that beautiful effect with ourselves when we show affection and love. The hormone oxytocin is released in response to giving and receiving compassion, enhancing feelings of security, trust, and calmness.

Self-compassion also helps us be more mindful of our well-being; it's like having a GPS for the body and soul. From regular exercise and healthy eating to avoiding harmful habits like smoking and excessive drinking, self-compassion empowers us to make choices consistent with our long-term health.

Instead of focusing on short-term pleasure, we can learn to shift toward a long-term perspective on our physical and mental wellness. We invest more time and energy into making decisions that will benefit us and our future selves.

Chapter Takeaways

- Self-compassion is a highly effective means of coping in healthier ways.

- Self-compassion is a powerful tool that can help individuals to improve their emotional well-being, build a stronger sense of self-worth, develop resilience, and improve their relationships and physical health.
- Having greater self-compassion makes you more tenacious and speeds up your recovery after experiencing negative emotions like shame, guilt, or anger.

Chapter 3
Embracing your Inner-Critic

"Too many people overvalue what they are not and undervalue what they are.

— *Malcolm S. Forbes"*

I know how challenging it can be to show yourself kindness, trust me. Activating the calming system can be a unique experience that may provoke resistance and complicated feelings. This is because it is very different from the more familiar threat-driven cycle many people are accustomed to. When first learning to practice self-compassion, it is common to experience an increase in negative thoughts. Do any of the following thoughts sound familiar to you:

"I don't have time for self-compassion. I need to focus on getting things done."

"Being too understanding toward myself means I'm not holding myself accountable."

"I don't deserve a break. I should just tough it out."

"If I'm not criticizing myself, I'll never improve."

"Being nicer to myself means I'm not taking things seriously."

"If I'm too kind to myself, I'll become a pushover, and people will walk all over me."

We all have those negative thoughts that creep into our minds and make us doubt ourselves. They tell us we're not good enough, that our goals are unattainable, and that our accomplishments don't matter. These thoughts might greet us in the morning as we look in the mirror, telling us how unattractive we are and how we're not good enough. They might pop up at work, telling us that we're not capable of handling the pressure and that we're invisible to others. And they might even influence our closest relationships, making us question whether we're truly loved and if our relationships will last. But here's the thing: these thoughts don't define us. We are so much more than the negative voices in our heads.

When it comes to practicing self-compassion, there may be times when it feels like you're climbing a mountain of insurmountable negative thoughts and feelings. But fear not; several strategies can help you overcome these barriers when learning to be kinder to yourself.

Cultivating Empathy and Compassion

One approach is to start by cultivating empathy for others and gradually working your way toward being more compassionate to yourself. It may be easier to show compassion for others before turning that emotion inward. Think of it like a warm-up before a big game. This tactic is like a stepping stone that helps you ease into feeling kindness toward yourself, transforming your inner critic into an inner friend.

Exercise

1. Start by setting aside some quiet time for yourself. Find a comfortable place where you can sit undisturbed for a few minutes.

2. Close your eyes and slowly try to let go of any thoughts or distractions by focusing on your breath. Take your time and keep your attention on breathing in and breathing out.

3. Now, bring to mind someone you care about. It could be a friend, family member, or even someone you don't know personally but admire. Imagine this person in your mind and try to feel empathy for them. Imagine what they might be going through, what they might be feeling, and what they might need.

4. As you focus on this person, feel compassion for them. Imagine yourself sending them love and support. Try to feel the warmth and kindness in your heart as you think of them. Focus on your bodily sensations. Where do you feel the warmth and kindness?

5. Once you have practiced empathy and compassion for someone else, bring your focus back to yourself. Remember that you are also human and have struggles and difficulties. Recognize your shared humanity with others.

6. As you focus on yourself, try to extend the same compassion and understanding to yourself that you were feeling for the person you were thinking of earlier. Focus on the bodily sensations you felt earlier and try to direct them toward yourself. Feel the warmth and kindness in your heart as you think of yourself.

7. Notice when you're being self-critical and try to reframe those thoughts in a more compassionate way. Challenge them by asking yourself where they're coming from and if they're true. Are they based on facts or emotions?

8. Take a moment to breathe deeply and release any tension you might be holding in your body. Allow yourself to let go of any distractions or worries and fully immerse yourself in the present moment. If it feels good, you can even release a sigh to help release any pent-up emotions. Take your time and allow yourself to relax and be in the present moment.

Imagining a Loved One's Perspective

Another approach is to put yourself in the shoes of a loved one. Imagine how they would perceive you and your situation. This can be much more effective than trying to generate feelings of self-compassion on your own. You can gain a new perspective on your situation and self-worth by seeing things differently.

Think about it, when you're feeling down, it's easy to get stuck in your head, and it can be hard to see the good in yourself. But, when you imagine how a loved one would perceive you, their love and concern for you can be a powerful reminder that you are worthy of kindness and compassion.

Exercise

1. Start by setting aside some quiet time for yourself. Find a comfortable place where you can sit undisturbed for a few minutes.
2. Close your eyes and focus on your breath. Take a few deep breaths in and out, and try to let go of any thoughts or distractions.
3. Bring to mind someone you love and trust. Imagine this person standing in front of you and try to picture their face clearly.
4. Imagine that you are explaining your current situation to this person and how you are feeling about it. Try to be as honest and open as possible.
5. Now, imagine how this person would respond to you. Feel their love and concern for you. Try to feel it in your body; in your heart. Imagine what they would say to you and how they would comfort you.
6. Take a moment to reflect on their response and how it makes you feel. Notice the warmth and kindness you feel. And let this feeling vibrate throughout your whole body.

Getting to the Root

You can get past your resistance to self-compassion if you take a good, hard look at the things that might be standing in the way. Self-compassion can be challenging to cultivate because of deeply ingrained, often learned, attitudes and emotions. In today's culture, where striving for perfection is highly valued, making a mistake may seem unacceptable. Complicating factors in relationships and interpersonal traumas can also teach us unconsciously that we aren't worthy of kindness and that love puts us in harm's way.

Beginning a self-compassion practice can feel strange initially, but that doesn't imply it's not doable. It's not like we're picking up an entirely new talent here. It eventually becomes second nature to treat ourselves like we would a trusted friend. Our natural instinct to fight or flee the situation makes us feel uneasy. When we make a mistake, our bodies react similarly under intense stress. We wage war on ourselves by verbally assaulting and humiliating ourselves to maintain some semblance of self-discipline or power. Or, we may become paralyzed, sinking into guilt and isolation.

Understanding the source of your negative thoughts and feelings can help you to take control and make them more manageable. It's essential to question the validity of these thoughts and feelings and to make an effort to change or challenge them.

By understanding the underlying causes of your negative thoughts and feelings, you can work toward making them more pliable. Thus, it will be easier for you to practice self-compassion.

Exercise

1. Find a comfortable place where you can sit in silence for a few minutes. It could be your living room, backyard, or car. Just make sure you won't be interrupted.
2. Now, close your eyes and focus on your breath. Take a few deep breaths in and out, and try to let go of any thoughts or

distractions. Let yourself relax and release any tension in your body.

3. Once you feel calm and centered, bring to mind a specific negative thought or feeling that prevents you from practicing self-compassion. It could be a thought such as "I'm not good enough", "This is stupid" or "I don't know if I can do this." Spend a few moments focusing on that thought or feeling and let yourself feel it fully.

4. Next, take a moment to examine where this thought or feeling came from. Ask yourself: "Is this thought or feeling truly my own, or are there external factors influencing it?" "Can I find ways to challenge or change this negative thought or feeling?" These questions are designed to help you understand the validity of your thoughts and feelings. It's important to realize that just because you have a thought doesn't mean you have to believe it or think it's true. Similarly, just because you have a feeling doesn't mean you have to act on it. The exercise helps you learn to challenge negative thoughts and manage complicated feelings.

5. Instead of trying to silence your thoughts or push your negative feelings away, try to accept and be with them. This is an integral part of self-compassion. Imagine yourself offering comfort to a loved one who is going through a difficult time. You wouldn't try to change their thoughts or feelings; you would simply be there for them and offer your support. The same applies to yourself. Accepting and being with your negative thoughts and feelings is not trying to change anything; you're simply being present and allowing yourself to feel and process whatever you're experiencing.

It can be easy to get caught up in negative thoughts and feelings that make us feel like we are not good enough. By understanding the origins of our inner critic and learning to be more compassionate toward ourselves, we can overcome these barriers and learn to practice self-compassion more effectively. Remember, self-compassion is not about ignoring or pushing away negative thoughts or feelings, but rather, it's about understanding and accepting them.

Chapter Takeaways

- When you first start experiencing your own kindness, you may feel resistance and experience an increase in negative thoughts.
- Easing into self-compassion by first focusing on the needs of others before directing that feeling toward oneself may be more manageable.
- By considering how a loved one would perceive you, you can shift your focus away from your perspective and gain a fresh and less biased viewpoint on your situation.
- By understanding and accepting negative thoughts and feelings, we can overcome these barriers and learn to be kinder to ourselves.

Chapter 4
Developing Loving-Kindness

The most powerful relationship you will ever have is with yourself.

— Steve Maraboli

Loving-kindness, also known as "metta" in Buddhism, is a powerful practice used for centuries to help individuals develop feelings of love and compassion toward themselves and others. It's a technique passed down from ancient Eastern spiritual traditions but has recently been adapted and studied in modern Western psychology. The purpose of this practice is to help us overcome the natural tendency to focus on our suffering and the suffering of those close to us and, instead, to open our hearts and develop a sense of interconnectedness with all beings.

Imagine being able to reduce stress, anxiety, and depression just by taking a few minutes each day to focus on love and compassion. That's the beauty of a loving-kindness meditation. Research has proven that regularly practicing this technique leads to many benefits, including lower levels of anxiety, stress, and depression.

Getting caught up in our problems and becoming trapped in a cycle of negative thoughts and feelings is easy nowadays. Loving-kindness meditation offers a way to break free from this cycle and develop a more compassionate and understanding perspective toward ourselves and others. It's an essential practice for anyone looking to improve their overall well-being. So, whether you want to reduce stress, improve your relationships, or feel more connected to the world around you, give loving-kindness a try and experience the benefits for yourself.

Loving-Kindness Meditation

The Loving-kindness meditation is a powerful practice that helps us tap into our innate capacity for compassion and kindness. It's important to remember that the words we use during the meditation are just tools, and the true focus should be on the feelings they induce. As we practice, the novelty of the words may start to fade, and that's okay. It's natural for our minds to wander, and the key is to bring our attention back to the emotion of loving-kindness.

This practice might sometimes feel awkward or frustrating (it's not uncommon for our minds to bring up negative emotions like anger or annoyance), but instead of getting caught up in these feelings, try to be gentle and compassionate with yourself. Accept whatever arises, and approach it with warmth and openness rather than judgment or shame.

It's also important to remember that this is not a one-time meditation, it takes time and practice to see the benefits, and the journey is what makes it all worth it.

Preparation

The first step in preparing for a loving-kindness meditation is to get comfortable. Sit with your feet flat on the floor, legs uncrossed, and back straight. Place your hands on your lap and take a moment to feel the connection of your body with the chair and the floor. Make yourself feel completely at ease.

Close your eyes if it feels comfortable. If it doesn't, you can gaze into your lap. Take a moment to observe your current state of sitting. It's like being a detective, investigating the present moment with curiosity.

As you tune in to your physical self and your breath, allow yourself to be present and aware, ready to accept whatever comes your way. You're going to be a true friend who is there for you every step of the way.

Calm your breathing and let go of any judgments or criticism. Just be. Take note of the inflow and outflow of your breath, like the tide coming in and going out. Feel the air passing through your nostrils and watch your chest rise and fall.

Now you're all set for your loving-kindness meditation journey, ready to explore the depths of compassion and kindness within yourself. So, take a deep breath, relax and let's begin.

Mindful attention

Once you're comfortable and in a relaxed state, it's time to focus your attention on your chest, close to your heart. This is where the magic happens. As you repeat to yourself in a soft and quiet voice, "Love. I pray that my heart will be filled with love," take a moment to feel the reverberation of the words in your chest.

Now, imagine someone or something you feel intense love and care for. It could be a loved one, a cherished pet, a favorite character from a book or show, or even a tree in your backyard.

Think about the warmth and happiness this person or thing brings you. Imagine the love and care radiating out of your chest and enveloping them.

Don't worry if you're unable to visualize or simply don't want to, it's ok, the feelings of love and kindness are the most important.

As you continue to repeat the phrase, "Love. I pray that my heart will be filled with love," allow yourself to fully immerse in the feeling of love and let it fill your heart and radiate throughout your body. It's like taking a warm bath for the soul.

This is a simple but powerful way to cultivate a feeling of loving-kindness toward yourself and others. Take a deep breath, relax, and let the love flow.

The cultivation of loving-kindness

As you focus on your heart, let a wave of compassion, kindness, and warmth wash over your entire being. Relax into the experience of these emotions. Now whisper to yourself slowly and repeatedly:

- May I always be brimming with loving kindness.
- May I be protected from all harm, both internal and external.
- May I be happy and contented.
- May all be well with my mind and body.
- May I find comfort and joy.
- May I forever rest in tranquility.

It may seem strange to speak kindly to yourself or even entertain such thoughts. Just keep repeating the sentences until you notice everything dissolving into the sensation of feeling safe and protected in this moment, the feeling of being content and happy in this moment, and the feeling of being complete in this moment.

Self-compassion is a practice not everyone feels immediately comfortable with. If you're having trouble, don't worry. It's normal, and it may take some time to get into the habit of doing this. So don't rush it; take your time.

Practicing kindness toward a loved one

Now think of someone you admire, appreciate, and respect, or perhaps someone who cares a great deal about you and only wants the best for you. It can be someone from the past or present, alive or who is no longer with us.

Imagine this person, and send them your best wishes. For example:

- I hope that you are protected from harm, both within and without.
- I hope that you are feeling good in both body and mind.
- I hope that you find peace and joy in life.

You may not even need words if you have a deep wellspring of compassion. This is your time for reflection, so feel free to adjust the practice as necessary.

Remember, sending love and kindness with an open heart is the most important thing. It's a small but powerful gesture of love.

Repeat the process with someone else in mind who is very important to you, for example your significant other. It's not about how many people you send loving-kindness to, but about the intensity, you send it with.

Extending kindness to a person who has no particular bias

Now, do the same thing with someone you don't know very well but don't dislike either. This could be a stranger you've seen on the street, on the bus, or in the hallway at work. Wish them well by sending these loving sentiments:

- I wish you to be brimming with loving kindness.
- I hope you are protected from harm, both within and without.
- I hope that you are feeling good in both body and mind.
- I hope that you find peace and joy in life.
- My wish is that you find rest and tranquility.

Sometimes, people may feel like they've lost touch with their capacity for kindness. But don't worry; it's never too late to reconnect with those feelings and start caring again. There's no need to rush; take your time cultivating a high-quality emotional response.

Extending compassion to someone who has upset or irritated you

Now, think of someone you've disagreed with or who has slightly annoyed you; it could be a colleague at work or a driver who cut you off on the road.

It's natural to have negative feelings toward someone who has irritated you but instead of holding on to those negative emotions, take this moment to extend compassion and kindness toward them.

It's not about agreeing with someone's behavior; it's about being able to treat them with respect and empathy.

Extending loving kindness to someone who has wronged you

As you focus on your heart area, think of someone who has wronged you. It could be someone who hurt you emotionally, betrayed your trust, or caused you pain in any way.

This might be the hardest part of this meditation, so be extra kind to yourself. Showing empathy for someone who has wronged us can be incredibly difficult. It's natural to feel anger and resentment toward the person who has hurt us, but holding on to these emotions can be a heavy burden to carry. It can weigh us down and prevent us from moving forward in our lives.

It's important to remember that empathy is not the same as forgiveness. Empathy means understanding and being able to relate to the feelings and experiences of another person. It doesn't mean that we excuse or justify their actions. However, by showing empathy, we can begin to understand why they might have acted the way they did and begin to let go of our anger and resentment towards them.

Now take this moment to extend compassion and kindness toward them.

Whisper to yourself slowly and repeatedly, "I wish you are protected from harm, both from inside and out", "I hope you feel good in body and mind", "I wish you find peace and joy in life", "I hope you find rest and tranquility."

Take a deep breath, relax and let the wave of compassion and love wash over this person. I know it's not easy, but showing compassion is a powerful tool that helps us heal and move on. It takes courage and self-awareness and is worth the effort in the end.

Now take a moment to recognize and appreciate what you have just done. Give yourself recognition for the incredible effort you made. Allow yourself to feel proud and give yourself the support and encouragement you need in this moment.

Putting out into the world a feeling of unconditional love

Now, expand your act of kindness outward to everyone and everything on Earth and beyond. Imagine a world filled with love and kindness, where everyone is protected, happy, and at peace.

It's like sending a love letter to the entire world, wishing everyone all the love, protection, and well-being. It's a way of spreading love and kindness to every corner of the world.

Practicing kindness and self-love toward oneself

Return your focus to yourself and allow loving kindness to fill your entire being. Breathe in peace and exhale peace. Be at peace with yourself and the world. Allow these emotions to permeate you while you softly and silently repeat to yourself:

- May I always be brimming with loving kindness.
- May I be protected from all dangers, both internal and external.
- May I be well in mind and body.
- May I find comfort and joy.
- May I forever rest in tranquility.

Finishing up

As you reach the end of your meditation practice, allow the warm fuzzies and feelings of love and kindness to fade away in their own time. Take a moment to come back to your breath, noticing the rise and fall of your chest and the sensation of the air moving in and out of your nostrils.

Take stock of your seating position, feeling the connection between your body and the chair, and the connection between your feet and the ground.

Notice the sounds around you, the gentle hum of traffic or birds chirping outside, and the natural ambiance of the present moment.

Take in the beautiful orange-brown hue of light you see against your eyelids, and when you're ready, gently open your eyes and focus on the present.

It's like coming back from a magical love-filled journey, feeling refreshed and rejuvenated, ready to take on the world with a heart filled with love and compassion.

Chapter Takeaways

- The practice of "loving-kindness" can help reduce our connection to painful mental states, allowing us to better weather their storms without being entirely overwhelmed.
- Loving-kindness involves showing love to yourself, people you love and admire, and even those who have annoyed or hurt you.

Chapter 5
The Map of Self-Compassion

You've criticized yourself for years, and it hasn't worked. Try approving of yourself and see what happens.

— Louise L. Hay

This chapter is designed to be a resource that you can come back to time and time again as you work to cultivate self-compassion in your life. The exercises and meditations included are meant to help you explore and strengthen your ability to be kind and understanding toward yourself. Whether you're new to self-compassion or looking for ways to deepen your existing practice, you'll find something that resonates with you here.

Take your time, explore the different exercises and meditations, and find the ones that work for you. Remember, self-compassion is a journey, not a destination, and with each step you take, you're one step closer to a more compassionate and kinder relationship with yourself.

Compassionate Body Scan

This exercise will focus on honing our physical selves through self-care. Too often, we neglect our bodies and only pay attention to them when they are in pain. Instead of wanting to impress others, self-care is about ensuring that we stay well and recognize the significance of our bodies' efforts on our behalf. Let's take a moment to appreciate the beautiful capabilities that our bodies possess and work on nurturing and valuing them. Let's begin.

Bring your attention to your current sitting position and make any necessary adjustments to focus completely on what's being said during the next few moments. Drop whatever has been stressing you out, worrying you, or otherwise weighing you down. Put both feet flat on the floor, keep your back straight but not rigid, loosen up your shoulders and facial muscles, and put your hands on your thighs or lap. You can close your eyes slowly.

Pause

It's easy to let our minds wander and leave our bodies behind. Mindful centering aims to bring us and our bodies back to the present moment. Take a few deep breaths to align your attention and body. Inhale through your nose, and exhale through your mouth, letting out a slow and leisurely breath. Repeat this process a few more times. As you release your breath, pay attention to how your body responds. This simple yet powerful practice brings harmony between your mind and body.

Pause

Now, observe the natural rhythm of your inhalations and exhalations as you let your breath move at its own rate. Take a few moments to focus on how it feels to breathe.

Short pause

It's natural for your mind to wander during this practice. If your thoughts stray, don't worry, it's normal. Without judgment, acknowledge the distraction and release it. Bring your focus back to your breath and continue with the practice. Remember, it's not about perfection but about being mindful and present in the moment.

Short pause

Let's look into your internal experiences now. Focus on the sensations you're currently experiencing. Take a walk through your body, starting at the top of your head and working your way down. As you scan through your body, take note of any areas that feel tense, relaxed, or neutral. For example, you may notice a tightness in your jaw or a knot in your shoulders or may notice a sense of calm in your chest or a feeling of lightness in your legs. Whatever you feel, don't try to change it, simply acknowledge it.

Short pause

Now, take a moment to evaluate your current mental state. Notice when you become aware of a thought and label it as "thinking." After you have labeled the thought, come back to your breathing.

Short pause

Get in touch with your feelings now. Don't worry about trying to interpret the origin of your feelings; simply say the word "feeling" as you're experiencing them and return to your breathing. Keep in mind that you aren't looking for how much or how little you can observe. The point is to pay attention to your internal experiences without judgment.

Short pause

Now let's focus on taking care of our physical health. We often only pay attention to our bodies when they are in pain instead of valuing and nurturing them when they are well. We should appreciate the amazing things our bodies can do for us and strive to improve our ability to care for ourselves. Let's give some thought to the incredible capabilities that our bodies currently possess and work on improving our ability to nurture and value them.

Pause

As you take your next breath, deliberately focus on your face—experiment with relaxing your facial muscles, starting with your eyebrows and jaw. Our heads are incredibly complex and powerful, allowing us to communicate, express emotions, eat, see, smell, hear, think, and taste. Take a moment to appreciate the hard work your facial muscles put in every day and allow them to rest and recover.

Short pause

Now, bring your attention to your neck and shoulders. If you feel any tension, try to release it with your next exhale. Our necks and shoulders often bear the weight of carrying heavy objects, and the strain of working at a computer and stress from our daily lives can also manifest as pain in these areas. Show gratitude and care for your neck and shoulders by taking a few deep breaths and letting go of any tension.

Short pause

Bring your focus to the chest area now. Notice how your chest rises and falls with each breath. Try listening to the sound of your heartbeat. The lungs and heart are vital for our energy system as they bring in oxygen and distribute it throughout the body. It is also the area where deep emotions such as happiness, sadness, joy, and grief originate. Take a moment to focus on this area of your body and pay attention to any sensations you may be experiencing.

Short pause

Bring your attention to your belly button now. Notice how your stomach moves with each breath. Feel your lower back move with each inhale and exhale. We often take for granted the work our stomachs do for us. Think about how your stomach processes food and provides energy for the rest of your body. Take a moment to appreciate and thank your stomach for all its hard work.

Short pause

Focus on your limbs now. How do your arms & hands feel? Are they cold, warm, or tired? Reflect on their sensations. Relax them and appreciate their capabilities. Think about the many times you use them during the day. Imagine how different your life would be without the ability to use your hands and arms.

Short pause

Take a deep, cleansing breath and direct your attention to your legs. Become aware of any sensations you might be feeling in your legs at this moment. Is there any tightness, discomfort, or fatigue?

Recognize the amazing things your legs are doing for you every single day. They have carried you through every step of your life's journey, supporting you and allowing you to move, explore, and experience the world around you.

Acknowledge the importance of taking care of your legs to ensure they are in top condition.

Short pause

Let's bring our attention to solely our feet. Notice where they make contact with the floor. Imagine breathing directly into your toes, and visualize yourself relaxing and massaging your feet with each exhale. Consider the feeling of taking responsibility for your own foot care. Your feet are the foundation of your body, and they work tirelessly to support you and the rest of your body every day.

Short pause

Take a deep breath and let it fill you up from head to toe; repeat this several times. Allow the air to reach every part of your body. Imagine it as an inward hug that you are giving yourself. Acknowledge and celebrate your body and all its features as you go through your day. Pay attention to how your body works as you use your hands to write or your feet to walk. Make a point to appreciate and be grateful for your physical self throughout the day.

Pause

When you are ready, slowly open your eyes. Take your time, and don't rush. Gradually start moving your fingers and toes, then your whole body, stretching gently and comfortably. Enjoy this wonderful feeling.

Self-Acceptance

In this meditation, we will work on self-acceptance and cultivating love and compassion for ourselves. We will explore how we can release negative thoughts or judgments about ourselves and learn to embrace our unique qualities and imperfections. Remember, self-acceptance is a journey and not a destination. Take a deep breath, and let's start.

1. First things first, let's get comfortable! Plant your feet firmly on the ground, and let your arms hang naturally by your sides. Place your hands on your lap, and bring your shoulder blades together. Lower your chin, so it's level with the floor, and raise your head so the crown faces upward. Take a moment to adjust your jaw and stomach for maximum comfort.
2. Now that you're settled, take a moment to appreciate the feeling of stillness. Take in the sensation of sitting in this thoughtful position at this precise time in this exact location. Give yourself a warm welcome to your practice, and acknowledge your desire to be here for yourself.
3. Next, let's focus on our breath. Pay attention to the sensation of the air entering and leaving your lungs. There's no need to control or alter your breath; just let it be as it is. Concentrate on your in and out breaths.
4. As you breathe, pay attention to where the sensation of breathing lands. You might feel the air entering and leaving your nose or the sensation of your chest and ribs expanding and contracting. Maybe you'll notice your stomach rising and falling. Just relax and focus on the ins and outs of your breath for a while.
5. As you focus on your breath, you may find random thoughts pop into your head. Don't worry, this is normal! Instead of trying to shut them out, let your thoughts pass through your mind one at a time. Recognize that these thoughts are just thoughts, and they do not define you as a person. Observe your thoughts without judgment and without attachment.

6. As you continue to breathe and focus on your thoughts, pay attention to any emotions that may arise. Take deep breaths in and out, and accept your feelings exactly as they are. Remember, all feelings are valid and encouraged in this practice.

7. Imagine yourself surrounded by a warm and loving light. This light represents the love and acceptance that you have for yourself. As you continue to inhale, imagine that light growing brighter and brighter, filling your body and mind with a sense of self-love and acceptance.

8. Take a moment to focus on all the things you appreciate about yourself, your strengths, your kindness, your determination, your courage, your ability to learn, your ability to grow, etc.

9. Check in with your posture, and see if it has changed at all. Tune in with your body, notice any sensations, and adjust anything that feels uncomfortable.

10. As you come to the close of this practice, take three more deep breaths in and out. Be present for each and every one of them. Remember, you have access to this state of being at all times, within yourself.

11. When you're ready, slowly open your eyes and take in your immediate surroundings. As you go about your day, strive to be present and conscious in all of your interactions.

Resolving Emotional Wounds from The Past

In this meditation, we will explore how faith can help us heal from past emotional wounds and find peace in the present moment. We will focus on the power of forgiveness, gratitude, and trust and how these elements can support us in our journey toward emotional healing.

Pain and suffering can lead to significant growth and personal development. Through these difficult experiences, we can learn and understand ourselves more deeply. However, it is essential to maintain a sense of hope and optimism to navigate these challenging times effectively. We can work toward healing and finding new perspectives by aligning our hearts, minds, and actions. Keep in mind that adversity often leads to personal growth and development.

By the end of this meditation, you will have a deeper understanding of the restorative power of faith and how you can use it to resolve your own emotional wounds.

- Find a comfortable position and start by focusing on your breath. Take a moment to settle into your body and let go of any tension you may be holding.
- Bring to mind any emotional wounds you may be carrying with you. It can be memories or feelings of hurt, betrayal, or disappointment. Acknowledge and accept these emotions without judgment.
- Imagine that you are holding each of these wounds in your hands. See them as physical objects, and feel how heavy and burdensome they are.
- Take a deep breath and exhale away any negative emotions or bodily sensations that may not be serving you. Paying attention to your breath can bring a sense of calm and tranquility to your mind and body. Let your thoughts drift effortlessly along with each exhale.
- Now, let's focus on the power of forgiveness. Imagine that you can forgive the person or situation that caused these wounds and feel the weight of the wounds begin to lift as you forgive.
- Next, we will focus on gratitude. Imagine that you are grateful for the lessons and growth that came from these wounds. See yourself becoming stronger and more resilient due to what you have gone through.
- Finally, let's focus on trust. Imagine that you trust in a higher power, whether it be a god, the universe, or your own inner guidance, to lead you toward healing and peace. See yourself letting go of the wounds and trusting that you will be guided toward what is best for you.
- As you continue to focus on forgiveness, gratitude, and trust, feel the emotional wounds begin to fade away. Imagine that

they are being replaced with light and peace. Take a moment to feel the peace and tranquility that comes with healing.

- Remember that healing is a process and the power of hope can help us through the difficult moments. Trust in yourself and the journey, and know that you are becoming stronger and more resilient with each step.
- When you are ready, take one more deep breath and open your eyes. Remember that the restorative power of faith is always available to you whenever you need it.

Cultivate Compassion

In this meditation, we will use the NEED technique to bring awareness to our thoughts, emotions, and physical sensations, as we focus on cultivating compassion toward ourselves and others. The NEED technique is a powerful tool to help us develop a deeper understanding of ourselves and the world around us by bringing awareness to our experiences in a non-judgmental way. During this meditation, we will use the four steps of Notice, Embrace, Examine, and Detach, to help us bring compassion to the present moment. Let's begin by finding a comfortable position, closing our eyes, and taking a deep breath.

Notice

As you take a deep breath, begin recognizing your thoughts, emotions, and physical sensations. Take a moment to acknowledge what is present in your mind and body.

You might notice your racing thoughts or a feeling of tightness in your chest. You may feel a knot in your stomach, or your shoulders may be tense. Whatever it is, observe it and acknowledge it. Like a detective on the case, you're gathering evidence of what's going on in your mind and body. By recognizing these thoughts, emotions, and physical sensations, we're setting the stage for the next steps of our meditation.

Embrace

The following minute will consist of taking a slow, deep breath and allowing yourself to be. As you exhale, imagine yourself blowing away any resistance to your thoughts, emotions, and physical sensations. It's like releasing a helium balloon into the sky, letting go of the string, and watching it float away.

Notice if there is any judgment or criticism you might have toward yourself or others. And let it be without trying to change or push it away. This step is all about embracing the present moment without trying to change anything.

Examine

Now take a closer look at your thoughts, emotions, and physical sensations. Observe them with curiosity and without judgment, like a scientist studying a specimen under a microscope. Ask yourself, what might be the underlying issue that is causing these thoughts, emotions, and sensations? It's like solving a puzzle, piecing together the clues to understand the bigger picture. This step is about understanding and gaining insight into your thoughts, emotions, and physical sensations.

At this point, we usually start to feel some strain. When we practice openness and curiosity with love, we can identify, grant permission, and inquire into the regions of our inner world that need care, cultivation, and nurturing, just like tending to a garden. We can reap a harvest of understanding and success by nurturing these parts of ourselves.

Detach

In this last step, we're going to detach from the experience by recognizing that it is not a part of the self but simply something that is happening in the present moment. Picture yourself stepping back and observing the experience from a distance, like watching a movie. You are a wise and loving observer who can see the situation clearly without getting caught up in it.

Try to bring an open heart and a sense of loving awareness without becoming too wrapped up in the situation. You want to prevent shifting into judgment and conviction, which will take you away from the disarming and curious state of mind that comes from simply sitting in natural awareness.

Take a deep breath and release all the tension from your body as you exhale. Imagine yourself freeing all the tension from your body like a balloon deflating. Take a moment to be with yourself and your compassionate intentions. Imagine yourself surrounded by a warm and loving energy and a sense of compassion. Allow this compassion to radiate outwards, enveloping yourself and those around you.

When you are ready, you can open your eyes.

Cultivating Joy in 8 Breaths

This guided meditation is a simple yet effective way to increase your overall well-being in just eight short breaths. Each inhale and exhale is associated with a single word to guide your focus and enhance the experience.

Remember, the 8 breaths in this exercise are merely symbolic and are not a strict requirement. You are free to take as many breaths as you need for each step.

1. Start with the inhale and focus on the physical act of breathing. Repeat the word "**breath**" to yourself and concentrate on the full cycle of inhaling and exhaling, and feel the sensation of air entering and leaving your body.
2. As you take a second breath, pay close attention to every sensation in your body. Be present in the moment and let your awareness permeate every cell. Take note of any good, painful, or neutral sensations you may be experiencing. Try not to modify your feelings and see what happens. This inhale is referred to as "**body**."
3. On the third breath, make a conscious effort to let go of any remaining stress, fatigue, or anxiety. Visualize it leaving your

body with each exhaled breath. This sigh of relief is referred to as "**release**."

4. With the fourth breath, send positive thoughts to yourself. Think kind and loving thoughts toward your brain and body. This is the "**love**" breath.

5. As you take the fifth breath, take stock of any cravings or aversions you may be experiencing. Acknowledge them rather than trying to suppress them. This breath is described as "**desires**."

6. The sixth breath is all about focusing on the present moment. Realize that this moment contains all the elements necessary for your happiness. There are an endless number of reasons to be happy and an infinite number of reasons to be sad right now. Thinking about where we want to focus can help us make better decisions. This breath is referred to as "**letting go**."

7. On the seventh breath, take a moment to marvel at the gift of life. Recognize the incredible value of the present momentary existence. This breath is referred to as "**alive**."

8. Finally, make the most of your eighth breath by fully appreciating the splendor of your inner and outer worlds. Relax and take it easy as you absorb the beauty of your surroundings. When we stop trying to control our surroundings and start living in the here and now, we realize that reality is breathtaking. Let's just relax and take it easy. This inhale is the epitome of "**beauty**."

Whether you have just a few minutes to spare or a whole hour, take the time to practice these eight breaths to elevate your happiness levels.

Chapter Takeaways

- **Compassionate Body Scan:** This guided meditation helps you to be more kind, accepting, and aware of your physical sensations. By focusing on different parts of your body, you'll learn to observe them without judgment and cultivate a sense of compassion toward yourself.

- **Self-Acceptance:** This meditation is designed to help you learn to accept yourself more fully. Through this practice, you'll come to terms with reality and develop a deeper understanding of your thoughts, emotions, and physical sensations.
- **Healing pain from the past:** This practice aims to release past pain and negative memories that may be holding you back from living in the present. It helps to create space for new experiences and reduce inner and outer conflicts.
- **Cultivate Compassion:** This four-stage process of becoming aware of ourselves, acknowledging that awareness, exploring it, and sitting with it, helps to cultivate a sense of compassion toward ourselves and others.
- **Cultivating joy:** This practice aims to develop a sense of joy and happiness. This guided practice is a quick and easy way to enhance your overall well-being in just a matter of eight breaths.

Chapter 6
Journey to the Core

You can't change the outside without changing the inside.

— *Yong Kang Chan*

Trauma is like a shadow that follows us wherever we go, shaping our thoughts, emotions, and actions without us even realizing it. It can be the source of our deepest pain and self-doubt, preventing us from living fulfilling lives. Unresolved traumatic experiences can contribute to negative self-talk, self-doubt, and feelings of worthlessness. These negative thoughts and feelings can make it challenging to be kind and understanding toward ourselves.

This chapter will guide you through the process of uncovering and healing past traumas and beliefs that may be holding you back from living your best life. We will delve into the powerful connection between past trauma and self-compassion and explore how healing past traumas can be the key to unlocking a life of greater happiness, self-acceptance, and inner peace.

Nurturing Your Inner-Child

You may have heard buzzwords like "inner child work," "shadow work," "childhood trauma," and "re-parenting" floating around lately, but don't let the trendiness fool you - these concepts are fundamental when it comes to our personal growth. They are an integral part of our being and play a crucial role in shaping our thoughts, emotions, and actions. Through inner child work, we can learn to heal the emotional wounds and unmet needs of our inner child and help it to grow into a strong, healthy, and well-rounded part of ourselves.

Imagine a young plant that was planted in dry, rocky soil and didn't receive enough water or sunlight. The plant will struggle to grow and likely be stunted and weak. Similarly, if we experience neglect or abuse during childhood, we may struggle to grow emotionally and develop negative behavior patterns or low self-esteem.

Just as a gardener would provide the right amount of water, sunlight, and fertilization, inner child work involves providing your inner child with the proper care by connecting with it in a healthy way and nurturing it through self-compassion. This process involves exploring your past experiences, addressing past traumas, and replacing toxic patterns with positive, nurturing ones.

As adults, we may think that our childhoods were normal and that our parents did the best they could. Childhood trauma can stem from various sources, not just abuse or neglect. Even seemingly innocent family dynamics can leave an imprint on our inner child.

We may not see how the stress and challenges of daily life, like balancing work and family, can affect a child's emotional well-being. But to a child, these situations can be traumatic and leave deep emotional wounds.

These wounds can then be carried into adulthood, affecting our thoughts, emotions, and behaviors, and even passed on to our children. Inner child work allows us to understand and heal these wounds and develop a healthy and loving relationship with ourselves and, subsequently, with others.

Exercise: Connecting with your inner child

- Before we start this meditation, remember that if at any point you feel the need to pause, go ahead and do so. Your experience is unique, and it's important to move at your own pace and be present in each moment. Take all the time you need.
- First, find a comfortable and quiet place where you can relax, focus, and won't be disturbed. Close your eyes and take a deep breath, let go of any distractions and let yourself be fully present in the moment.
- We often believe that our childhood story ends when we become adults, but it doesn't necessarily. Our inner child remains alive within us, carrying the essence of who we once were. No matter how loving or unloving our upbringing was, the child within us holds a special place in our hearts and in our memories.
- Now go back in time and imagine yourself as a child. Take yourself to a specific age and place that holds special memories. Take a close look at your inner child. How old are they? Notice their physical features, attitude, body language, and overall demeanor. What is your first impression of this child?
- As you focus on this image, pay attention to any emotions or thoughts that come to mind. These may be related to specific memories or experiences from your childhood. Notice your emotions without judging them and return to focusing on your inner child.
- Once you've identified these emotions or thoughts, initiate a conversation with your inner child. Ask them how they're feeling today and what's on their mind. Listen attentively to their response, allowing them to express themselves freely. Show your inner child that they are heard and valued, creating a safe and nurturing space for them to share.
- Now, thank your inner child for their honest answers and offer them comfort and reassurance. Tell your inner child that you understand and are there for them.

- Spend some time in silence, allowing your inner child to express anything else they might want to share. Keep listening attentively and try to understand their perspective. This is your inner child's chance to speak, and it's important to be a good listener.
- When you feel ready, tell your inner child you will work on meeting their needs in healthy ways as an adult. Remember that your inner child is a part of you and needs your love and care. Say goodbye to your inner child and give them a loving embrace.
- Slowly come back from the depths of your internal world and open your eyes.
- Take a moment to journal about your experience. Write down any emotions, thoughts, or insights that came up during the exercise. This will help you reflect on what you've learned and connect with your inner child in the future.

Exercise: Healing Childhood Trauma

Our childhood experiences shape who we are and can affect us profoundly. In this exercise, we'll look within ourselves to face and heal any pain from our past. This journey of self-discovery will help us turn our struggles into strengths and move forward confidently.

Step 1: Setting the Scene

Begin by closing your eyes and taking a few deep breaths. Imagine yourself standing in front of a large door. This door represents the entrance to your healing journey. Take a moment to notice any feelings or sensations that come up for you as you stand in front of this door.

Step 2: Creating Your Guide

Next, imagine that you are creating a guiding companion to help you on your journey. This guide can take any form you like - it could be a person, an animal, or even an object. Consider what qualities you would like your companion to have - for example, are they kind and supportive or strong and protective? Once you have a clear image of your guide in your mind, give them a name and welcome them to your journey.

Step 3: Entering the Healing Forest

With your guide by your side, imagine walking through the door and entering a beautiful forest. This forest represents the different parts of yourself you will be exploring on your journey. Notice the different trees and plants you see – each represents various aspects of your past experiences.

Step 4: Meeting Your Inner Child

As you continue to walk through the forest, you come across a small child sitting on a tree stump. This child represents your inner child - the part of you that experienced the trauma. Notice how the child feels - are they scared, sad, or angry? Take a moment to acknowledge their feelings and let them know you are here to support them.

Step 5: Facing Your Trauma

As you continue to walk through the forest with your guide and inner child, you come across a clearing. In the center of the clearing is a representation of the traumatic event you experienced. It could be a person, a place, or an object. Take a moment to notice how you feel as you approach this representation. Your guide is there to support you and your inner child as you begin to process and work through your trauma.

Step 6: Finding Inner Strength

After some time, you begin to notice that you feel stronger and more empowered. This is because you have faced your trauma and can now move forward. Imagine that you are now leaving the clearing and walking deeper into the forest. As you walk, you come across a tree that represents inner strength. Take a moment to sit underneath this tree and imagine that its strength is flowing into you.

Step 7: Emerging from the Forest

After some time, you come to the edge of the forest. You can see a bright light shining in the distance. This light represents your healing and growth. Take a moment to say goodbye to your guide and inner child, and thank them for their support on your journey. As you step out of the forest, take a moment to notice how you feel - you may feel lighter, more at peace, and more in control of your emotions.

Step 8: Reflecting on your Journey

Take a moment to reflect on your journey and write down any insights or revelations that came up for you during the exercise. Remember that healing is a process and that taking your time is okay. You can revisit this exercise whenever you need to and continue to work through your trauma in a supportive and creative way.

Unveiling the Higher Self

Many of us go through life feeling lost, disconnected, or unfulfilled without realizing that the answers we seek lie within ourselves. Imagine a wise and all-knowing version of yourself who is always by your side, whispering words of wisdom in your ear. Your higher self is always speaking to you, but we are often reluctant to listen to it. Your higher self is the part of you that is in tune with your deepest desires, your highest potential, and your ultimate purpose. It is the voice within that guides you toward your passions and your destiny. It is the compass that points you in the direction of true fulfillment.

Exercise: Unlocking the Secrets of the Soul

- Take a deep breath and close your eyes. Imagine a bright, warm light at the center of your chest. This is the light of your higher self, shining bright and strong.
- Now, focus your attention on the area of your chest. Pay close attention to your senses and keep track of any changes that may indicate that you've made a connection. You might feel a sense of calm, warmth, expansion, or connection. These are all signs that you're on the right track.
- Next, try to locate the source of the feeling. Imagine that your higher self is an actual being you can communicate with. Imagine that you're sitting across from it, looking into its eyes. Imagine that simply being in its presence makes you feel better.
- Now, speak to your higher self. Ask it for guidance, advice, or insight. You might get an idea, a feeling, a symbol, or just a gut feeling as an answer. Don't worry if the solutions you're looking for don't come to you immediately. Sometimes, the answers come in a dream or at a time when you're more emotionally prepared to hear them.
- As you speak to your higher self, pay attention to the way your body feels. Does it feel light and relaxed, or heavy and tense? This can be a sign of whether the advice you're receiving is in alignment with your true self or not.
- When you feel like the conversation is over, thank your higher self for its guidance and open your eyes. Take a moment to reflect on what you've learned, and write it down in your journal. If you feel like the exercise helped, repeat it over the course of several days.
- Remember, connecting with your higher self is not always easy, but it is a journey worth taking. With practice, you'll get better at recognizing the signs of a connection and trusting the guidance you receive. So, keep an open mind, stay patient, and enjoy the adventure!

Receiving validation from within

Validation is essential for our emotional well-being; it helps us feel seen, heard, and understood. But, seeking validation from others can be a futile and never-ending quest, as we are constantly changing and evolving, and what we need to feel validated might also change. That's why it's essential to learn to seek validation from within.

Your higher self is the part of you that is connected to your inner wisdom; it knows what is best for you and what you genuinely need to feel fulfilled. It's the voice inside of you that guides you toward your purpose and helps you navigate through life's challenges. But it's important to note that listening to your higher self takes time and practice.

The following exercise can help you start the process of seeking validation from within.

Exercise

1. Take a few deep breaths and find a quiet place where you can sit comfortably without any distractions.
2. Close your eyes and bring your awareness to your breath. Lay your hands on your heart, on your stomach, or simply by your side.
3. Take a moment to reflect on a time in your life when you sought someone's attention, approval, or acceptance. Pay attention to the initial thoughts that arise and allow yourself to acknowledge them without judgment or dismissiveness.
4. Ask yourself what you would have wished this person would've told you. What kind of validation were you looking for?
5. When you have the answer, ask yourself the following question: Why do I need their approval to feel important, support to feel supported, and love to feel loved?
6. Repeat this question several times, and be open to receiving different answers.
7. Once you have a clear answer, take a moment to reflect on it.

8. Ask yourself: "How can I give myself the validation I need right now?" "What does my body need?" "What can I do to improve my mental and physical health and well-being?"

9. Listen to your inner wisdom and take the necessary steps to give yourself the necessary validation. If the answers to these questions did not come to you immediately, give it time and keep practicing this meditation.

By regularly practicing this exercise, you will build a deeper connection with your higher self and learn to rely on its guidance for validation.

A letter of Support from Your Higher Self

We all have moments in life when we feel lost, alone, or unsupported, and it can be hard to find the motivation and confidence to keep going when we're in a difficult place. That's why it's crucial to have a source of support that we can always turn to, and that source of support is ourselves.

Our higher self is the part of us that is always there to guide and support us; it knows what is best for us and what we need to hear in difficult times. But sometimes, it can be hard to listen to its guidance, especially when we're feeling down. That's why I want to introduce you to an exercise that can help you get the support you need from your higher self.

Exercise

1. Take a piece of paper and a pen, or open a word document on your computer.

2. Imagine that you have an imaginary friend who is loving, accepting, kind, and caring and who would never judge you or cause you any harm. Think of this person as someone who can see you exactly as you are right now, including the parts of yourself you don't like or keep hidden. Consider how your friend feels about you and how much they love you despite your flaws. This friend understands that you are human and is gracious and forgiving. This wise companion knows that the

sum of your experiences, as countless as they may be, have shaped you into the person you are now.

3. Now, write a letter from this loving person's perspective about how you take care of and talk to yourself. Imagine someone who has boundless compassion, approaches you, and offers advice. How would your friend express their sympathy for you, especially in light of the anguish you experience due to your own severe self-criticism? And if this person were to offer advice about what you should do to improve your life, how do you think they would do so in a way that exemplified unconditional love and kindness?

4. When you're finished, put the letter away and read it the next time you feel down. Take in the words that your friend has to offer. Keep the letter somewhere safe, where you can refer to it whenever you need a reminder of your inner strength and wisdom.

Remember, this exercise can be repeated as often as you need; it's a great tool to help you connect with your higher self and receive the support you need. And remember, you have the inherent right to be loved, connected, and accepted.

Chapter Takeaways

- Trauma can shape our thoughts, emotions, and actions without us realizing it, leading to negative self-talk, self-doubt, and feelings of worthlessness.
- Inner child work is an approach to help heal past traumas and develop a positive relationship with oneself, which in turn improves relationships with others.
- Our higher self is the inner guide that always supports us and knows what's best for us.
- We can learn to nurture and support ourselves without needing external validation by connecting with our inner child and higher self.

Chapter 7
Compassion in Relationships

"You never really understand a person until you consider things from their point of view...until you climb inside of their skin and walk around in it".

— *Harper Lee*

The journey of self-compassion is a never-ending one, and when we think we have mastered it, we realize there's another layer to uncover. By being more compassionate toward ourselves, we come to realize that we have not been truly able to extend compassion unconditionally to others in the past. It's like we've been walking around with a blindfold on all this time. We couldn't see the good in ourselves, let alone in others. But when we start treating ourselves with kindness and understanding, our blindfold is lifted, and we see the world in a whole new light.

As we become more self-compassionate, we are filling ourselves up with the resources we need to give back to others. We feel better about ourselves and have more energy, patience, and kindness to offer to those around us.

This chapter will explore how self-compassion and being compassionate to others are interconnected. We will discover that compassion and empathy are essential for building stronger relationships and fostering a more peaceful and harmonious world. We will learn how to put ourselves in others' shoes, understand their struggles and joys, and offer them the same kindness and understanding we have learned to offer ourselves.

Compassion In Conflicts

Conflict is an inevitable part of life. Whether with a friend, family member, or coworker, we all have to navigate disagreements and differences of opinion from time to time. But, when conflicts arise, it's easy to get caught up in our own emotions and react in ways that can escalate the situation and cause further harm. And let's face it; we've all been there.

But when we approach conflicts and disagreements with compassion and understanding, we can avoid becoming entrenched in our own positions and instead seek to understand the other person's perspective.

Compassion can be a powerful tool in this process, allowing us to step back, observe the situation without judgment, and approach the conflict with an open mind and a compassionate heart.

Self-compassionate people have a more positive and understanding attitude toward themselves and others regarding mistakes and failures. They understand that everyone is human and imperfect and don't resort to criticizing or blaming themselves or others for errors. Instead, they have a "cushion" of kindness and a selfless motivation to improve themselves. This allows them to take responsibility for their actions and apologize when necessary.

It is natural for people to become defensive and blame others when problems arise as a way to avoid self-criticism and self-loathing. However, self-compassionate people are more self-aware and approach these situations differently by treating themselves and others with the same empathy and kindness. This makes it easier for them to admit their mistakes and work toward finding solutions.

Here are some tips on how to practice compassion for others in conflict situations:

1. **Listen actively:** When you are in a conversation with someone with a different opinion or perspective, try to listen actively to what they have to say. Don't think about how you will respond, and avoid interrupting or dismissing their thoughts. Instead, keep asking questions to gain a deeper understanding of their viewpoint.
2. **Avoid getting defensive:** It's natural to feel defensive when someone challenges our beliefs or opinions. Getting defensive distracts you from feeling hurt or shamed and shifts the focus to the faults of the other. See if you can become aware of defensiveness and create a moment for yourself to nurture any difficult feelings. When you've acknowledged and validated your feelings try returning to the conversation with an open mind.
3. **Find common ground:** Find areas of agreement and shared values. This can help to build a foundation of understanding and respect.
4. **Stay open to learning and be curious:** Approach the conversation with a mindset of learning and growth rather than trying to convince the other person of your point of view.
5. **Practice empathy:** Try to put yourself in the other person's shoes and understand where they are coming from. Empathy helps to build understanding and connection.
6. **Keep perspective:** Remember that people's opinions and views are often shaped by their experiences and backgrounds, and try not to take things personally.
7. **Respectful disagreement:** It's okay to disagree, and it's important to respect other people's opinions, even if they differ from yours.

The Need for Healthy Boundaries

Healthy relationships are built on a foundation of compassion. However, compassion alone is not enough; it must be balanced with healthy boundaries, or it can lead to co-dependency and neediness.

When we enter into a committed relationship, it can be easy to fall into the trap of thinking that our partner should fulfill all of our emotional needs and alleviate all of our concerns. We may even begin to feel responsible for their happiness and become overly invested in their emotions and well-being. This is co-dependency, a form of compassion gone awry.

Similarly, neediness is another sign that compassion and boundaries are not balanced in a relationship. Needy individuals may fear rejection or abandonment and may become overly dependent on the validation and attention of others. They may struggle to form a sense of self-worth and look to others to validate their worth.

Both co-dependency and neediness can lead to unhealthy dynamics in relationships, where one person becomes overly invested in the emotions and well-being of the other and struggles to set and maintain healthy boundaries to take care of themselves.

It is important to remember that compassion and healthy boundaries are not mutually exclusive. We can have compassion for others while also being aware of our needs and limits. This means learning to practice self-compassion, being kind and understanding toward ourselves, and learning to set and maintain healthy boundaries. It involves saying "no" when necessary, setting limits on the time and energy we spend on others, and taking care of our physical, emotional, and mental well-being.

Compassion is vital to healthy relationships but must be balanced with healthy boundaries. By learning to practice self-compassion and to set and maintain healthy boundaries, we can foster healthier and more fulfilling relationships.

Strategies to Set Healthier Boundaries

Align your boundaries with your values: Consider your personal values and beliefs when setting boundaries. Use them as a guide to help you determine what you are and are not willing to tolerate in your relationships.

Clarify your intentions: Think about what you want to achieve by setting boundaries. This can help guide your decision-making process and ensure that your boundaries align with your goals.

Evaluate existing relationships: Take the time to reflect on your current relationships and identify any areas where you may need to set boundaries. This can help you assess your relationships' health and make necessary changes.

Recognize relationship differences: Different relationships may require different boundaries. For example, you may have stricter boundaries with a close friend than with a co-worker. It's important to understand that boundaries are not one-size-fits-all and should be tailored to each individual relationship.

Practice and patience: Setting and maintaining boundaries can be challenging and may take time and practice. Be patient with yourself and understand that it's a process that requires effort and dedication.

Speak up respectfully: Communication is key when it comes to setting boundaries. Clearly and respectfully express your boundaries to those in your life. Be confident and assertive in your delivery to ensure that your boundaries are understood and respected.

Pay attention to changes: Relationships can change over time, and it's important to consider these changes. Be mindful of any shifts in your relationships and adjust your boundaries as needed to maintain a healthy balance.

Hold your ground: Maintaining healthy boundaries requires consistency and commitment. Be firm in upholding your boundaries, even in difficult situations. Remember, you have the right to set boundaries that protect your mental and emotional well-being.

Compassion in the World

In today's world, we face a growing number of conflicts and divisions between individuals, groups, and societies. From political tensions to social divisions, it can often feel as though the world is becoming more and more polarized.

It has become easy to fall into the trap of judgment and suspicion toward those different from us. We surround ourselves with like-minded individuals, avoid being challenged or exposed to new perspectives, and feel stronger and more certain because of it. However, we must let go of the illusion that certainty is a sign of strength. True strength lies in our ability to be vulnerable, curious, and humble.

By letting go of our need for affirmation, validation, and approval, we can disentangle ourselves from the idea that we always have to be right. Instead, we can focus on understanding others and how to empathize with them. In doing so, we can build trust and cooperation between people, groups, and societies with different opinions and perspectives.

When we are willing to let go of our judgments and assumptions about others and practice compassion, we open ourselves up to a world of possibilities. We let go of judgment and invite curiosity; we learn to see things from different angles and challenge our beliefs, leading us to a deeper understanding and connection with those around us.

While judgment closes us off to new ideas and perspectives, curiosity opens us up to discovery and exploration. It allows us to see the nuances and complexities in a situation and challenges us to question our assumptions. It's in this state of curiosity that real growth and understanding can occur.

So how do we put this into practice? By following the core principles of self-compassion and applying them to others.

Self-awareness: Self-compassion helps increase self-awareness, allowing you to recognize and understand your thoughts and emotions without judging them. We have become better at identifying and labeling our emotions, understanding how they affect our thoughts and behaviors, and recognizing the triggers that lead to negativity. This can help you approach conversations more clearly, better understand the complexity of the other person's thoughts and emotions, and prevent you from getting defensive.

Emotional regulation: Self-compassion helps to regulate emotions, which can be beneficial when encountering people with different opinions or perspectives. It allows you to have a calm and rational conversation with them rather than getting into a fight or argument. It also helps you to understand where they are coming from and to find common ground.

Perspective-taking: Self-compassion fosters an attitude of perspective-taking, which can be helpful when interacting with people with different opinions or perspectives. It allows you to understand where the other person is coming from and empathize with their viewpoint, even if you disagree with it. It also helps you to communicate your perspective more effectively, as you can anticipate and address any potential points of contention.

Avoiding perfectionism: Self-compassion helps to avoid perfectionism, the need to be right all the time and always be understood. You become more open to new ideas, and less likely to get stuck in your own point of view. This mindset can help with feeling less attacked and increase the willingness to learn from the other person.

Self-forgiveness: Self-forgiveness allows you to let go of any guilt or negative feelings you may have toward yourself for not understanding or agreeing with others. By forgiving yourself, you can approach the situation with a more open and curious mindset rather than feeling offended or angry. This can lead to more productive and understanding conversations and help reduce any stress or tension you may feel. By being more self-forgiving, you will also be more understanding of the other person and their mistakes and limitations.

Chapter Takeaways

- Practicing self-compassion gives us more energy, patience, and kindness to offer to others, resulting in more positive relationships.
- Approaching conflicts with compassion and understanding leads to a more positive and productive outcome.
- Self-compassion and healthy boundaries are crucial to fostering positive and fulfilling relationships.
- We can build trust, cooperation, and understanding with people and groups that have different opinions and perspectives by using the core principles of self-compassion.

Chapter 8
Self-Compassionate Parenting

Raising little humans can be one wild ride. It's a mix of heartwarming moments and head-scratching moments. You'll find yourself being patient one moment and being tested the next. You'll feel like you're on top of the world when you see your child achieving something new and feel like the worst parent in the world when you can't get them to do something. As much as we love our children, the reality is that parenting can be incredibly challenging. We feel exhausted, anxious, and worried and may feel like we are not doing a good job or living up to our expectations. Fortunately, the practice of self-compassion can help us navigate these challenges and find a way to parent with joy, happiness, and exuberance.

Self-compassionate parenting is about shifting our focus from constantly trying to fix or change ourselves and nurture ourselves so we can be the best parents possible. It is about recognizing that we are all doing our best and need to care for our well-being to support our children better.

This chapter will explore the concept of self-compassionate parenting and how it can help us to be happier, more patient, and more understanding parents. We will discuss the importance of self-care, self-compassion, and self-kindness in parenting and provide practical tips and strategies for incorporating these practices into our daily lives. We will also explore the benefits of self-compassionate parenting for both parents and children, including improved physical and mental health, reduced stress, and better parent-child relationships.

The Challenges of Parenting

One of the most significant challenges of parenting is the constant self-evaluation and criticism that parents place on themselves. This self-judgment can manifest in feelings of inadequacy, low self-esteem, and frustration toward both ourselves and our children.

Some of us might criticize ourselves for not being the perfect parent, making mistakes, or not having all the answers. We feel the need to have the perfect home, the perfect family, and the perfect children. But deep down, we all know that perfection is unattainable, and the constant pursuit of it can lead to feelings of disappointment and failure.

It's important to remember that parenting challenges are typical and expected and that every parent goes through difficult times. Building a sense of community with other parents who understand the trials and tribulations of parenting can provide powerful support and alleviate feelings of isolation, guilt, and blame. We can receive genuine support and understanding by opening up about our struggles and finding someone who can truly empathize with us.

Parents must understand that their own struggles are often reflected in their children's struggles. By prioritizing self-care, they can better provide the support and guidance their child needs.

The Importance of Self-compassionate Parenting

Studies have shown that parents who practice self-care and self-compassion have better physical and mental health, are more confident in their parenting, and have more positive interactions with their children. Self-compassion is associated with lower levels of parental depression and parenting stress, as well as reduced fatigue. By treating themselves with kindness, understanding, and forgiveness, parents set an important example for their children, showing them how to be compassionate and resilient in the face of life's challenges.

One of the key benefits of self-compassionate parenting is that it can help children develop a strong sense of self-worth. When children see their parents treating themselves with kindness and understanding, they learn that they too are worthy of love and respect. This can help them build a positive self-image, which is essential for their emotional and mental well-being.

Another great benefit of self-compassionate parenting is the development of resilience. Children who see their parents handling difficult situations with compassion and understanding are more likely to learn how to cope with their own challenges in a healthy and effective way. They learn that it's okay to make mistakes and that they can bounce back from setbacks.

Self-compassionate parenting can also help children build solid and meaningful connections with others, which is essential for their social and emotional development. When children see their parents treating themselves and others with kindness and understanding, they learn the importance of empathy and compassion in their own relationships.

Practicing Self-Compassion in Parenting

Teaching children the concepts of self-compassion can help them navigate the challenges of life with more joy and happiness. Parents can play an essential role in helping their children develop self-compassion by setting an example and providing guidance.

Here are some tips for introducing the concepts of self-compassion into parenting and helping children develop a self-compassionate mindset.

- Have your child think about a time when they were hard on themselves or felt guilty about something. Ask them how they would feel if a friend came to them with the same problem. Encourage your child to talk about how they would respond and what advice they would give to their friend.

- Explain to your child that it's normal to experience strong emotions such as sadness, frustration, or disappointment. Provide reassurance that these feelings are valid and acceptable and avoid dismissing how they're feeling in that moment. Offer encouragement, such as saying "I understand that you're upset. It's okay to feel that way. Sometimes things don't go as we plan."

- Teach your child the value of forgiveness, both for themselves and others. Show that mistakes are a natural part of life and that letting go and moving forward is important. Express empathy, for example, by saying, "I know you didn't mean to break that. Accidents happen, and it's okay."

- Have your child practice talking to themselves in a supportive and friendly tone, using the advice they would give to a friend. Encourage them to repeat a positive affirmation or mantra that they come up with, such as "I am doing my best" or "I am worthy of love and kindness."

- Acknowledge and praise your child when they show compassion towards themselves. Emphasize how important it is to be kind and understanding. Offer words of encouragement like "I'm proud of you for being so understanding and giving yourself another chance." This helps build their self-compassion and reinforces the idea of treating oneself with love and kindness.

- Practice self-care together. Encourage your child to take time for activities they enjoy, such as reading, sports, or music.

- Help your child to develop a daily self-compassion practice. Encourage them to spend some time each day focusing on the positive aspects of their life and themselves. You can even make a habit of listing some of the things you appreciate about your child before bedtime and letting them do the same thing.

Remember that self-compassion is an ongoing practice that requires consistency and patience. But with your guidance, your child will learn to be kinder and more understanding of themselves and be better equipped to handle life's challenges with more joy and happiness.

Chapter Takeaways

- Self-compassionate parenting is about nurturing ourselves, recognizing that we are all doing our best, and prioritizing our own well-being in order to better support and guide our children.
- Self-care and self-love are essential for effective parenting as it helps parents to understand and address their struggles.
- Self-compassionate parenting has many benefits for both parents and children, such as better mental and physical health, more positive interactions, and the development of self-worth, resilience, and connections with others.
- With proper guidance, children can learn to be more compassionate toward themselves, making them more resilient and better able to handle life's challenges with happiness and joy.

Chapter 9
The Nurturing Power of Self-Care

"Our sorrows and wounds are only healed when we touch them with compassion."

— *Buddha*

When you're feeling like you're about to go off a cliff and into the depths of despair, self-care can be an excellent intervention tool that quickly pulls you back up. Contrary to popular belief, self-care is more than just bubble baths and face masks; it's about taking care of yourself on a deeper level. It's about nourishing your mind, body, and soul. It brings you joy and peace just because you're making time for yourself and engaging in activities that make you happy.

A Guide to the Practice of Self-Care

Self-care is essential for our overall happiness and mental health. It is the process of taking an active role in protecting our well-being and is an essential aspect of self-regulation and self-compassion. In the past, it was believed that our brains were hardwired and unchangeable, but recent studies have shown that the brain is malleable and can be rewired.

One way to move past our primitive 'fight-or-flight'-response is by prioritizing self-care and making a conscious decision to adopt two alternative responses: empathy and action. Empathy is the ability to understand and share the feelings of others, and action is taking steps to address the problem and improve the situation.

Experts recommend the following three ways to take care of yourself:

1. Refuel, refresh, and get ready to act. Taking a break from the constant stimulation of the news, social media, and other distractions is important. By switching off the TV, logging out of social media, and disabling alerts and push notifications, you can improve your concentration and spend some time in peace and quiet.
2. Learn to identify the signs that indicate you need to take care of yourself and act accordingly. Taking care of yourself can positively affect your relationships with others. For example, when you need to ask a coworker to cover for you or a babysitter to watch the children. It is important to listen to your body and mind, and recognize when you need rest, relaxation, or self-care. Remember that in the end, taking care of yourself not only benefits you but also improves your relationships with others.
3. Create a self-care checklist with a wide variety of items that you can choose from. A bubble bath or a midday phone call with a friend are just two examples of the many self-care activities you can choose from. If you're on the verge of burnout, you should have this list prepared in case you suddenly find yourself unable to think of any solutions. We will further dive into this later in this chapter.

Admitting you need help is a courageous act of self-care. Remember, self-care is an ongoing process, and it's important to take your time. By prioritizing self-care, you can rewire your brain to adopt more positive and effective responses to stress and adversity.

The Need for a Self-Care Strategy

A self-care plan is a personalized blueprint for taking care of yourself physically and emotionally. It's a roadmap that guides you through difficult times, providing you with the tools and resources to navigate life's challenges.

Creating a personalized self-care plan is a preventative measure that can help you proactively address the stresses of life. By taking the time to consider your needs and the resources you have at your disposal, you can create a plan that will guide you through difficult times with ease. Only you know the limits of your stress and the extent to which you have support at your disposal, so a self-care plan tailored to your unique needs is essential.

Having a plan in place for self-care removes the need for impromptu decision-making when facing adversity. From the perspective of awareness, this allows you to act instead of react. Having a strategy in place might help you feel less stressed and more in command of your life. Telling others about your plans before you seek help makes the process much simpler. This can be helpful in case of emergency or worst-case scenario.

A self-care plan can also help you stay on track. It will be much less of a struggle for you to stick to your self-care plan and avoid giving in to the excuse-making trap. If you and your self-care friend are serious about preventing isolation, planning regular get-togethers can help. You can share the duty of helping one another and checking in with one another regularly. This can be a great way to remind yourself that you're not alone in your struggles and that there are people who care about you and want to help.

Creating a self-care plan can also help you avoid falling into negative patterns and equip you with the necessary skills to handle stressful situations and challenging life events. It provides you with a set of coping mechanisms that can help you manage and navigate these difficult times, keeping you grounded and in control.

Creating Your Self-Care Plan

Self-care is essential for our overall well-being, but creating a personalized self-care plan can be overwhelming. Follow these five steps to create a self-care plan tailored to your individual needs and start taking care of yourself proactively and intentionally.

Step 1: Take a look at your current habits

Before making your self-care plan, taking a good look at where you are now is essential. Reflect on the strategies you currently use to deal with life's demands. Do you go for a walk to relieve stress or tend to withdraw from your friends and family? Do you have a glass of wine after a tough day at work or take a long bath to relieve tension? Write down an honest inventory of your positive and negative coping strategies. This step will help you identify any harmful habits and your existing self-care practices.

Step 2: Identify your self-care needs

Now that you better understand your current habits, it's time to think about what you value most in your day-to-day life. Make a list of all your physical, mental, emotional, and professional needs. A good self-care plan should consider all areas of well-being. This step may be a real eye-opener, you may discover you're already meeting your physical needs, but you're neglecting your emotional needs.

Here are some examples of different types of needs to help you along:

Physical Needs

- Eating a balanced diet
- Getting enough sleep
- Regular exercise

- Managing chronic health conditions
- Preventive health care, such as regular check-ups and screenings
- Taking medications as prescribed

Mental Needs

- Managing stress
- Finding time for hobbies and leisure activities
- Practicing mindfulness or meditation
- Engaging in creative activities
- Learning new skills
- Accessing mental health care as needed

Emotional Needs

- Building and maintaining positive relationships
- Finding a sense of belonging and connection
- Expressing emotions in a healthy way
- Finding healthy ways to cope with difficult emotions
- Setting boundaries and assertively communicating needs

Professional Needs

- Building a career or pursuing further education
- Setting and achieving personal and professional goals
- Networking and building relationships in the industry
- Continuously learning and developing new skills
- Finding work-life balance
- Finding job satisfaction and fulfillment

Step 3: Write down practices that support your needs

It's time to decide which self-care activities will help you meet your needs. Consider asking yourself questions like 'What activities bring me joy?' 'What helps me feel energized?' 'What makes me feel fulfilled?'

'What's helped me cope with difficult moments in my life?' Write down the self-care practices you plan to do daily and those you'll only do once in a while. For example, you'll want to eat healthy daily, but you may only schedule dinner with a friend once a week.

Step 4: Fit your activities into your schedule

Now it's time to find pockets of time throughout your busy day to incorporate these practices. Remember, self-care isn't selfish; it's an act of kindness to yourself. Instead of jamming all sorts of activities into your day, start small. Add one to two activities into your routine each week, and before you know it, you'll have a full-fledged self-care routine. Prioritize the practices you need and value the most, and evaluate how they're helping you improve yourself.

Step 5: Remove any barriers

It's time to let go of any negative habits that are getting in the way of your self-care plan. Replace them with self-care practices, and don't be afraid to ask for help from your friends or family members. Sharing your self-care plan with a supportive network can help you overcome obstacles more easily. And remember, self-care is an ongoing process, so update and adapt your plan as needed.

Claiming Your Healing Time

Incorporating self-care into our daily routine is crucial for maintaining our physical, mental, emotional, and spiritual wellness. It's easy to get caught up in the hustle and bustle of daily life and neglect our own needs. But just like a car needs fuel to function, we, too, need to take care of ourselves to keep going.

Think of the low fuel warning light on your car's dashboard. When it comes on, you know you have a limited amount of time before you'll have to stop and refuel. The same is true for our well-being. We must pay attention to the warning signs that we're running low on energy and take steps to refill our tanks before it's too late.

Try being completely honest with a trusted friend or loved one about your needs, whether it's a need for space or support. Sharing your thoughts and feelings with someone you trust can alleviate some of the stress preventing you from taking care of yourself. Trust me, when you open up and share your thoughts and feelings with someone you trust, you will find an understanding and supportive listener who will be there for you.

Let's revisit the "low fuel" signal on your car's dashboard. When your warning light turns on, it's important not to ignore it. There's also no need to panic or waste energy worrying since you probably still have about 30 miles worth of gas left. If you feel like you're reaching a point of exhaustion or burnout, it's important to immediately take action and reach out to people you trust before reaching a boiling point. Address minor issues before they become bigger problems.

Don't be afraid to reach out and ask for what you need. It's in our nature to be helpful and kind to one another. We're wired to have empathy and feel good when we do good things for others. That's why acts of kindness happen all around us every day. So, it's safe to assume that plenty of people in your life would have been more than happy to lend a helping hand if only they were asked. The problem isn't their willingness to help; it's our hesitance to ask.

Self-Compassion at Work

Let's face it; when it comes to our job performance, we can be our own harshest critics. It's like a switch flips as soon as we step into the office - all the self-compassion and forgiveness we practice in our personal lives go out the window. We put ourselves under a microscope and expect nothing short of perfection - handling all the pressure and stress like a pro, never missing a beat, and always on our A-game. But even at work, we must remind ourselves to be kind and recognize that we all make mistakes and have weaknesses.

In this book, we have delved deeply into strategies for cultivating self-compassion, equipping you with the tools to apply them in the workplace. To remind you of some strategies to help achieve this, here are four ways to cultivate self-compassion at work.

1. **Prioritize self-care:** It's easy to neglect our needs when busy, but taking care of ourselves is essential for our well-being. Make time for activities that nourish your body, mind, and spirit, such as eating well, going for a walk, and connecting with colleagues. And don't be afraid to take a break when you need one.
2. **Embrace your imperfections:** We all have moments of self-doubt and feelings of imposter syndrome, but it's important to remember that everyone experiences these things. Recognize that you are not alone in your struggles and that your imperfections do not define you.
3. **Be kind to yourself:** It only makes things worse when we're hard on ourselves. Instead, consider yourself a friend in need and offer yourself the same encouragement and support you would give to someone else.
4. **Ask for help:** We often feel that we should be able to handle everything on our own, but that is just not realistic. Remember that it's okay to ask for help and that others will often be happy to support you.

Chapter Takeaways

- Self-care is not just about pampering yourself; it's about taking action to improve your overall well-being on a physical, mental, emotional, and professional level.
- A self-care plan is necessary to address and manage stress and adversity proactively.
- Self-care strategies equip us with healthier coping skills and avoid falling into harmful habits.
- We must stop being extra hard on ourselves at work and acknowledge that we can make mistakes and will always have weaknesses.

Chapter 10
Transforming Your Mindset with Affirmations

"Most unhappy people need to learn just one lesson: how to see themselves through the lens of genuine compassion and treat themselves accordingly."

— *Martha Beck*

Thoughts are powerful things, shaping our perception of the world and influencing our actions and decisions. Our thoughts are like a lens through which we view the world, and they can either limit or expand our possibilities.

How we think about ourselves, our abilities, and our circumstances can profoundly affect our reality. For example, if we believe we can succeed in a particular endeavor, we are more likely to take the necessary steps to achieve that success. On the other hand, if we believe we are not capable or that success is not possible, we are less likely to take action.

Our thoughts also shape our emotional state. Positive thoughts can lead to happiness, motivation, and contentment, while negative thinking leads to sadness, hopelessness, and frustration. Our emotions, in turn, influence our behavior and actions.

It is important to note that thoughts aren't simply random musings; they are closely connected to our beliefs and experiences, and our past shapes them. We can learn to change negative thoughts and ideas to create a new reality that aligns with our goals and values.

Affirmations are a powerful tool to help us align our thoughts and comments with our intentions and manifest the life we desire. They help purify our thoughts, restructure our mindsets, and can help make us believe anything is possible. With regular use, affirmations can help us to achieve our goals, build self-confidence and ultimately, live our best lives.

How Do Affirmations Work?

Our thoughts are connected to specific paths in our heads. Just like electricity travels through circuits, our thoughts travel through these paths in our brains. When we think the same thing over and over, it gets easier for our brain to think that way, and it becomes a habit. This happens even if the thought is not a good or correct one. Instead of allowing our heads to overflow with negative thoughts, we can actively choose to counter those thoughts with positive affirmations.

Great thinkers, successful businesspeople, and spiritual leaders have used affirmations for centuries. They are a simple yet powerful tool that can help us overcome limiting beliefs, build self-confidence, and even manifest our wildest dreams. But affirmations aren't just for the elite few, they're for anyone who wants to improve their lives and achieve their goals.

Affirmations work by reprogramming our subconscious mind. Our subconscious mind is the part of our brain that controls our automatic thoughts and actions. It is responsible for many of our habits and beliefs and is often the source of negative thoughts and self-doubt. By repeating affirmations, we are giving our subconscious mind new information to process and new views to adopt.

This can help to replace negative thoughts and ideas with positive ones.

Making sure the affirmations you're using resonate with you, is very important, as this will help you connect to them emotionally. To build belief, try visualizing the affirmation as if it's already happened, and imagine yourself living it. When negative thoughts come up, counteract them with positive affirmations. Over time, this can help change negative patterns of thinking.

Affirmations are most effective when they are specific, personal, and written in the present tense. For example, instead of saying, "I will be successful," it's more effective to say, "I am successful." This helps to create a sense of immediacy and makes the affirmation feel more natural.

If you're initially skeptical about positive affirmations, don't worry - you're not alone. Many people are hesitant to try affirmations, but in many cases, that has to do with a misunderstanding of their purpose. It's important to understand that positive affirmations are not a standalone solution for achieving our desires. Simply repeating affirmations alone will not bring about change.

To fully benefit from affirmations, they must be accompanied by intentional action and effort. Affirmations serve as a catalyst for setting our intentions, but it's up to us to put in the work to make those aspirations a reality. Consider affirmations as the starting engine - they provide the initial push, but it's up to us to keep moving towards our destination.

How to Practice Affirmations

- **Choose your affirmations:** Select affirmations that resonate with you and align with your goals and values. Make sure they are specific, personal, and written in the present tense. You will find a list of self-compassion affirmations below that you can personalize and make your own.
- **Write them down:** Write your affirmations on paper or in a journal. Having them written down can help make them feel more natural and increase their effectiveness.

- **Repeat them regularly:** Repeat your affirmations to yourself multiple times a day. It's best to repeat them when you first wake up and before bed, but you can also repeat them throughout the day as needed. It may take some time to notice a change, so be patient and keep at it.
- **Say them with conviction:** When you repeat your affirmations, say them with conviction and believe in them. Speak them out loud or in your mind with enthusiasm and emotion.
- **Visualize:** Visualize yourself already having achieved the things you want to achieve while you are saying the affirmations.
- **Track your progress:** Keep track of your progress by noting any changes you notice in your thoughts, feelings, or behaviors. This will help you see the impact of your affirmations and keep you motivated to continue.

Self-Compassion Affirmations

1. I am kind and compassionate toward myself.
2. I treat myself with the same care and understanding I would offer to a good friend.
3. I am worthy of love and acceptance, including my own.
4. I am allowed to make mistakes and learn from them.
5. I am patient and understanding with myself.
6. I accept my imperfections and celebrate my strengths.
7. I am worthy of self-care and self-nurturing.
8. I am strong and capable of handling difficult emotions.
9. I trust my inner wisdom and intuition.
10. I give myself permission to feel and process my emotions.
11. I am enough, just as I am.
12. I let go of self-criticism and embrace self-compassion.
13. I am open to learning and growing from my experiences.
14. I am not defined by my past mistakes or failures.
15. I am deserving of a fulfilling and happy life.
16. I am kind to myself in my thoughts and actions.

17. I am grateful for my unique qualities and talents.
18. I am willing to forgive myself for past mistakes.
19. I trust in my ability to heal and grow.
20. I am worthy of respect and dignity, including my own.
21. I choose to focus on my positive qualities and strengths.
22. I am compassionate toward myself in times of stress and struggle.
23. I am patient with my progress and trust the journey of self-improvement.
24. I am not alone in my struggles, and seek support when needed.
25. I am proud of my accomplishments and recognize my efforts.
26. I am open to learning from my mistakes and taking responsibility for my actions.
27. I am kind to myself and practice self-care regularly.
28. I recognize my worth and value as a human being.
29. I choose to be gentle and understanding with myself.
30. I am willing to let go of self-doubt and trust in my abilities.
31. I am capable of change and growth.
32. I am compassionate toward myself and others.
33. I am grateful for the opportunity to learn and improve.
34. I am worthy of a fulfilling and satisfying life.
35. I practice self-compassion daily and strive to be my best self.

Conclusion

The journey of self-compassion is a powerful and transformative one. By learning to be kind, gentle, and understanding with ourselves, we unlock the full potential of our minds and hearts. Through the practice of self-compassion, we learn to embrace our humanity, accept our flaws and imperfections, and live life to the fullest.

We come to understand that our self-worth is not dependent on our achievements or failures, but rather on our inherent value as human beings. We all have value, and we all deserve kindness, no matter what. Self-compassion allows us to release the grip of negative self-criticism and replace it with a sense of calm and interconnected acceptance, turning anguish into happiness.

This book has explored the various aspects of self-compassion and how it can be applied in our daily lives. We began by explaining the concept of self-compassion and recognizing self-criticism. We delved into practical exercises and meditations to help us cultivate self-compassion in our daily lives. We explored how self-compassion can help us be more resilient, cope with stress and anxiety, improve our relationships, and find meaning and purpose in our lives. We also saw how it can help us overcome perfectionism and be more creative. By learning to be more compassionate with ourselves, we have developed more compassion for others and, in the end, are able to create a more compassionate world.

Learning self-compassion is like learning a new language. Just like you wouldn't become fluent in a new language by simply acknowledging its existence, you won't develop self-compassion without consistent practice. To develop self-compassion, it's important to keep paying attention to the things you tell yourself, especially when times are rough.

Self-compassion is a life-changing expedition that requires determination and hard work, but the rewards are beyond measure. This book serves as your compass, providing the tools and guidance needed to embark on a journey of self-discovery and growth. By practicing self-awareness, self-care, and compassion, you will not only transform your relationship with yourself, but also the way you interact with the world around you. Embrace the journey with open arms and a curious spirit and I'm sure you will be pleasantly surprised at where it might take you.

Bibliography

Abblett, M. (2022, January 10). *Mindful Parenting: Meet Your Inner Critic with Self-Compassion.* Mindful. https://www.mindful.org/mindful-parenting-meet-your-inner-critic-with-self-compassion/

Baulch, J. (2022, February 8). *Why is Self-Compassion so Hard Sometimes?* Inner Melbourne Psychology. https://www.innermelbpsychology.com.au/why-is-self-compassion-so-hard-sometimes/

Breines, J. G., & Chen, S. (2012). *Self-compassion increases self-improvement motivation.* Personality and Social Psychology Bulletin, 38(9), 1133-1143.

Breines, J. G., & Chen, S. (2013). *Self-compassion and well-being in China: An examination of the mediating role of mindfulness.* Self and Identity, 12(1), 78-98.

Center for Mindful Self-Compassion. (2020, November 18). *What is Self-Compassion?* CMSC. https://centerformsc.org/learn-msc/

Chowdhury, R. B. M. A. (2022, September 12). *What Is Loving-Kindness Meditation?* (Incl. Scripts). PositivePsychology.com. https://positivepsychology.com/loving-kindness-meditation/

Coelho, S. (2022, September 7). *The Benefits of Self-Compassion.* Psych Central. https://psychcentral.com/blog/practicing-self-compassion-when-you-have-a-mental-illness

Colasacco, E. (2022, January 11). *Befriend Your Body: A Compassionate Body Scan. The on Being Project.* https://onbeing.org/blog/befriend-your-body-a-compassionate-body-scan/

Cratsley, R. F. (2023, January 3). *A Guided Meditation for Healing Through Hope.* Mindful. https://www.mindful.org/a-12-minute-meditation-for-healing-through-hope/

Davenport, B. (2022, August 26). *Follow This Self-Love Meditation Script To Treat Yourself With Compassion.* Mindful Zen. https://mindfulzen.co/self-love-meditation/

Davis, W. (2020, October 21). *Self-Compassionate Parenting.* Postpartum Support International (PSI). https://www.postpartum.net/self-compassionate-parenting/

Definition and Three Elements of Self Compassion | Kristin Neff. (2020, July 9). Self-Compassion. https://self-compassion.org/the-three-elements-of-self-compassion-2/

Germer, C. K. (2009). *The mindful path to self-compassion: Freeing yourself from destructive thoughts and emotions.* Guilford Press.

Gilbert, P., & Proctor, S. (2006). *Compassionate mind training for people with high shame and self-criticism: Overview and pilot study of a group therapy approach.* Clinical Psychology & Psychotherapy, 13(6), 353-379.

GoodTherapy Editor Team. (n.d.). *Self-Compassion.* https://www.goodtherapy.org/learn-about-therapy/issues/self-compassion

Hardy, J. (2021, June 17). *How to Practice Loving-Kindness.* Lions Roar. https://www.lionsroar.com/how-to-practice-loving-kindness/

Hendershot, C. (2022, March 18). *Meeting Difficult Emotions with Compassion.* Grand Rapids Center for Mindfulness. https://www.grandrapidscenterformindfulness.com/meet-difficult-emotions-with-compassion/

How to Practice Loving Kindness Meditation. (2020, February 11). Verywell Mind. https://www.verywellmind.com/how-to-practice-loving-kindness-meditation-3144786

Jones, C. (2023, January 10). *A 15-Minute Meditation for Self-Acceptance.* Mindful. https://www.mindful.org/a-15-minute-meditation-for-self-acceptance/

Just a moment. (n.d.). https://yogainternational.com/article/view/guided-meditation-for-self-love/

Kabat-Zinn, J. (2022, October 4). *This Loving-Kindness Meditation is a Radical Act of Love.* Mindful. https://www.mindful.org/this-loving-kindness-meditation-is-a-radical-act-of-love/

Kramer, J. (2021, November 8). *The benefits of self-compassion and how to cultivate it for yourself.* Centres for Health and Healing. https://cfhh.ca/blog/the-benefits-of-self-compassion/

Kuyken, W. (2022, January 18). *Sparking Joy: A Mindfulness Practice for Everyday.* Mindful. https://www.mindful.org/sparking-joy-a-mindfulness-practice-for-everyday/

Leary, M. R., Tate, E. B., Adams, C. E., Batts Allen, A., & Hancock, J. (2007). *Self-compassion and reactions to unpleasant self-relevant events: The implications of treating oneself kindly.* Journal of Personality and Social Psychology, 92(5), 887-904.

MacBeth, A., & Gumley, A. (2012). *Exploring compassion: A meta-analysis of the association between self-compassion and psychopathology.* Clinical Psychology Review, 32(6), 545-552.

Maldonado, M. (2021, November 16). *A Guided RAIN Meditation to Cultivate Compassion.* Mindful. https://www.mindful.org/a-guided-rain-meditation-to-cultivate-compassion/

Mangotich, H. S. T. (2020, October 15). *When Self Compassion is Hard.* Psychotherapytoronto. https://www.psychotherapyinthecity.com/post/when-self-compassion-is-hard

Medcalf, A. (2020, February 18). *IS SELF-COMPASSION THE SECRET TO A HAPPY RELATIONSHIP?* Abby Medcalf. https://abbymedcalf.com/is-self-compassion-the-secret-to-a-happy-relationship/

Megginson, M. (2022, February 3). *Why Self-Compassion Is Key to a Better Relationship.* The Center. https://www.thecenterportland.com/why-self-compassion-is-key-to-a-better-relationship/

Mental Health and Self-Care. (n.d.). Priory. https://www.priorygroup.com/blog/mental-health-and-self-care

Neff, K. D. (2003). *The development and validation of a scale to measure self-compassion.* Self and Identity, 2(3), 223-250.

Neff, K. D., & Germer, C. K. (2013). *A pilot study and randomized controlled trial of the mindful self-compassion program.* Journal of Clinical Psychology, 69(1), 28-44.

O'Brien, E. (2022, March 10). *Why Is It So Hard to Practice Self-Compassion?* Yoga Journal. https://www.yogajournal.com/lifestyle/why-is-it-hard-to-practice-self-compassion/

O'Leary, W. (2021, December 13). *7 Self-Compassion Reminders for Parents of Kids Who Are Struggling.* Mindful. https://www.mindful.org/7-self-compassion-reminders-for-parents-of-kids-who-are-struggling/

Parker, T. (n.d.). *Self-Compassion In Relationships.* http://thrivingrelationships.org/cultivate-compassion/self-compassion-in-relationships/

Redd, K. (2021, February 18). *7 Concrete Ways Self-Compassion Can Improve Your*

Marriage. Marriage Advice - Expert Marriage Tips & Advice. https://www.marriage.-com/advice/relationship/self-compassion-can-improve-your-marriage/

Ribeiro, M. B. (2022, August 13). *What Is Compassion Meditation? (+ Mantras and Scripts)*. PositivePsychology.com. https://positivepsychology.com/compassion-meditation/

Salzberg, S. (2022, January 19). *Why Loving-Kindness Takes Time: Sharon Salzberg*. Mindful. https://www.mindful.org/loving-kindness-takes-time-sharon-salzberg/

Staff, M. (2022, July 6). *A Guide to Practicing Self-Care with Mindfulness*. Mindful. https://www.mindful.org/a-guide-to-practicing-self-care-with-mindfulness/

Suraliya, S. (2022, December 2). *5 Life-Changing Benefits of Self-Compassion*. Your Mental Health Pal. https://yourmentalhealthpal.com/benefits-of-self-compassion/

The hidden benefits of self-compassion. (n.d.). https://www.betterup.com/blog/hidden-bene-fits-of-self-compassion

Tusa, S. (2020, July 28). *Joy Is a Radical Act. Tricycle: The Buddhist Review*. https://tricy-cle.org/article/joy-meditation/

What is Self-Compassion? (2016, January 1). GoStrengths! https://gostrengths.com/what-is-self-compassion/

Why Is Self-Compassion So Hard for Some People? (n.d.). Greater Good. https://greater-good.berkeley.edu/article/item/why_is_self_compassion_so_hard_for_some_people

Get Your Ebook Stop Limiting Yourself
+ Reduce Stress in 1 minute [video]
+ Printable Gratitude Journal

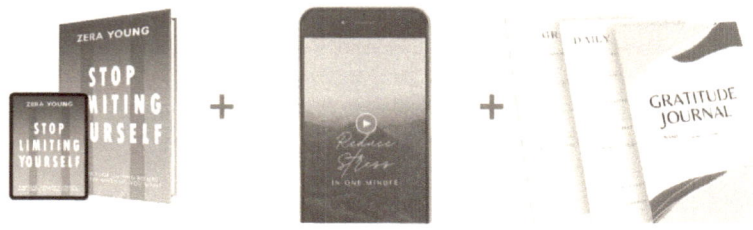

Scan the QR code below to claim your free bonuses
——————— OR ———————
visit gifts.zerayoung.com/bundle

Unleash your true potential and choose to live your best life!

✔ Free e-book: Stop Limiting Yourself. Stop doubting your potential and learn to recognize your self-limiting beliefs!

✔ Free meditation video: Reduce your stress levels in one minute with this powerful breathing exercise.

✔ Printable Journal: Print out your daily and monthly Personal Gratitude Journal for positive manifestation and improved self-confidence!